THE SEARCH

FOR

DYNAMIC HEALTH

CHARLES R M BOOTE

Filament Publishing
14, Croydon Road
Waddon, Croydon
Surrey CR0 4PA
United Kingdom
+44 (0) 20 8688 2598
sales@filamentpublishing.com

www.filamentpublshing.com

Printed by Antony Rowe Ltd, Eastbourne
Front cover design - Simon Greatbach. Zippa Communications

ISBN 0-9546531-9-X

The comments and recommendations in this book <u>do not</u> constitute any form of medical or professional advice, nor are they meant to be a substitute for the personal advice or counselling of a general practitioner or qualified health professional.

When purchasing dietary/nutritional supplements to support the maintenance of good health, it is important to appreciate that the companies marketing them, <u>do not</u> sell their supplements on the basis of curing or preventing disease. Dietary/Nutritional Supplements are <u>not</u> medicine. Dietary/Nutritional Supplements should be taken with a healthy well-balanced diet and are not a substitute for it.

Whilst the producer has taken all reasonable steps to ensure the accuracy of the information contained in this book, it is provided on the understanding that the author is not liable for any inaccuracies therein. The information and opinions in this book are for informational purposes only. Neither the publisher nor the author will be liable for any loss, injury, or damage allegedly arising from any information or suggestion in this book.

The statements and comments made in this book are the result of research undertaken by the author and many scientific and medical references are included. The author has relied in particular on the following publications and recommends them for further reading: "The Optimum Nutrition Bible" by Patrick Holford, Founder of the Institute of Optimum Nutrition, London; Institute for Natural Products Research – "Natural Supplements: A Desktop Reference" by Dennis J. McKenna, Ph.D., Editor-in Chief; The Antioxidant Revolution by Dr. James F. Balch published by Sound Concepts Inc. of Orem, Utah, USA and 8 Million-copy Best Seller – America's #1 Guide to Natural Health – "Prescription for Nutritional Healing" by Phyllis A. Balch, CNC and James F. Balch, M.D..

CONTENTS

FOREWORD

I have been involved in a number of things in my life from playing competitive sports, to a career in the Territorial Army, to being involved in several different types of businesses. Whilst I took a keen interest in looking after my health in my 20s and 30s, it was always in support of my other activities. But an early indication of my inherent interest in health was my choosing Biology as one of my A Level subjects at school, even though it would be of little help towards my chosen profession, accountancy.

After I left school I continued playing rugby football for 4 years until a car crash put paid to that. Although I was told I would have arthritis in my knees, which suffered badly in the crash, by the time I was 40, I was determined to get back to competitive sport even though rugby was off the agenda. My physiotherapist, who was a tower of strength in that period of rehabilitation, was under contract with the local 1st Division Football Team. He worked hard to get me back to full throttle again and did a great job. He told me the importance of exercise and nutrition to build my strength and stamina and help prevent arthritis. So, after a 4-year lay-off from all sports and back to full strength, I took up squash and played competitively for the next 8 years or more. As you will know competitive squash is one of the most energetic, stamina-draining sports you can come across and it is surprising to me that my legs stood up to the strain so admirably; thanks to the good advice and treatment I had received from my physiotherapist! I should also add that I am forever grateful to the surgeon who did such an excellent job after the accident.

Looking back it is amazing to me that my focus changed so quickly from recovering from my accident to all the issues surrounding full-blown competitive squash. This made me study nutrition more thoroughly, not only to protect my knees but also to improve my overall fitness and performance.

While still in my 20s, it had become clear to me that what I ate could make a positive contribution to my sports performance – would I have the stamina to win my match next Saturday, especially if my team's promotion to the next division at the end of the season depended on it? What was the point, I asked myself; of doing all that training if I didn't ensure my food intake was the best and most appropriate fuel I could take in? Ever since I left school I have always taken a multi-vitamin supplement plus extra b-vitamins for energy before a match or serious exercise.

As time marched on and it was time to retire from competitive sport, my interest in nutrition accelerated and I became an Associate Member of the Institute of Optimum Nutrition in London. I started to think about how I could stay fit and healthy – hence the reason for the name of this book – Search for Dynamic Health. I was concerned about doing what I could to keep away from disease; I had those nagging doubts, as so many people do, when I saw some of my friends die in their 50s, which I felt sure, in one way or another, could have been avoided at least in some of the cases. Quite frankly, I was determined to find out what could be done to help prevent fate holding so much sway over our lives on this earth. I knew that genetics play their part but usually only to a relatively small degree and it was becoming clear to me that simple lifestyle and nutritional choices on a daily basis were by far the most significant factor in achieving Dynamic Health. I was going to make sure that I found out all I could in order to achieve Dynamic Health for the rest of my life and the lives of my family. Part of the results of my research was my decision to take specific extra nutrition to support my damaged knees, especially after 8 years of competitive squash. I am pleased to say, 35 years on, that I have no signs whatsoever of arthritis.

I believe there are few people who wouldn't want to "Look Good, Feel Good, Perform Better, Keep Away from Disease and Die Young as Late as Possible!" That is what I call Dynamic Health. That is certainly what my family and I want to enjoy! As far as I am concerned, life on this planet is far too short not to do simple and reasonable things on a daily basis to achieve and maintain Dynamic Health. To me the issue is not just wanting to live longer, which is a natural instinct built into mankind – it's not wanting to spend the last 15 years of my life as a "creaking gate", not being able to see properly or in a wheel chair, or even both, <u>and</u> be dependent on others! I want to be active to the day I die and go out like a light bulb when the heart muscle has run its course. I don't want someone turning down my dimmer switch just because I'm 70 and then turning it down further when get to 80! I want to die young, with all my faculties, as late as possible.

What my research has uncovered is that there is an abundance of relatively new scientifically and clinically proven information out there, which most people have little or no knowledge of, which can help us achieve and enjoy Dynamic Health. The aim of this book is to impart to you some of this new and significant knowledge in the hope that it helps you and your family.

To me the most significant issue concerning health, which my research has turned up, is the change that is taking place in informed sections of the medical world from the principle that <u>germs cause most diseases</u> to the principle that <u>many diseases result from an imbalance that weakens the body</u>. Of course there are some microbes that are harmful, whether the body is balanced or not, such as the TB bacteria and Aids virus. However, even in those cases the severity of the illness is inversely proportional to the state of the body's internal environment and defence mechanism. Maintaining a balanced body in terms of nutrition, exercise, and lifestyle habits is critical to obtaining and maintaining Dynamic Health throughout our lives.

In my quest for the keys to enjoying Dynamic Health, I have watched how the years have caught up with people, some of whom I have known, but not seen for decades. Some had aged much faster than others and others had aged rapidly over only a few years. I kept asking myself why there were such differences between people; of course the lifestyle habits they had been indulging in often gave me a clue! My investigations also indicated that some were more knowledgeable on health matters than others and, as a result, usually more proactive towards their health, especially when it came to nutrition.

I have also observed how lifestyle habits such as smoking have taken their toll on some people at a relatively young age, whether visually or due to illness or premature death. The challenge that many people face in today's more sedentary world is that smoking that one cigarette or eating that one hamburger or bag of crisps won't kill you today! Indeed, smoking and eating hamburgers and crisps every day for a week won't kill you! But that damage accumulates little by little over time until some part of our body capitulates to the relentless onslaught throughout our lives as our bodies get more and more out of balance. Sooner or later, the statistics show that we are likely to become trapped in a diseased body often for years and even decades. For, you see, an out of balance body doesn't necessarily lead to a death sentence, but to a degraded existence, which I'm sure is not what most people want!

Another key development in the knowledge of the medical world over the last 15 years is that a major cause of imbalance in the body is Oxidative Damage caused by Reactive Oxygen Species or molecules left over from our metabolic processes and from stress and pollution and many other sources. A major reason for oxidative damage occurring at a faster rate in our bodies than is necessary is the significant lack of fruits and vegetables in our diets. Fruits and vegetables provide the anti-carcinogenic cocktail on which our bodies have evolved over time and which they need on a daily basis in order to stay in balance. We abandon that cocktail at our peril! Indeed, it is now known that there are over 300 plant chemicals that have clinically proven capabilities to protect the human body and keep it in balance.

Another concern I had, which is shared by most people, especially the Baby Boomers, was that I didn't want to age any faster than I had to! I soon discovered that ageing, as well as many diseases, is due considerably to Oxidative Damage to the cells and DNA in our bodies and is therefore inextricably linked to maintaining Dynamic Health. What is now conclusively proven is that today's foods are decidedly lacking in the nutrients we need and also that we often eat the wrong foods. To help prevent unnecessary Oxidative Damage occurring all over our bodies and to keep them in balance, it is now scientifically proven that Antioxidants, to a substantial degree, are the answer. Did you know that our bodies produce Antioxidants from the day we are born and that if we didn't have any Antioxidants in our bodies from birth, we would be dead in 3 days! That's how important they are to obtaining and maintaining Dynamic Health!

What I was also interested to know was where doctors fit into all of this. Most general practitioners/family doctors will agree that they are in the <u>disease</u> business, not the <u>health</u> business. In the western world we usually go to the doctor when we are ill; much less do we go when we want advice on keeping healthy. What we are talking about here, enjoying Dynamic Health, is helping us keep away from the Doctor, and, unfortunately to say, also from our infected hospitals, which I'm sure you agree is a worthy cause! At least what our enjoying Dynamic Health can do is to relieve our overstretched National Health Service in the UK, which has a mountain to climb in the next 30 years as it copes with all the Baby Boomers, now aged 40 to 58, as they start entering old age.

Another issue that struck me, on which I can now speak from experience, is that you can enjoy Dynamic Health every minute of every hour of every day, of every year. What else in life can you enjoy for so much of your time, which is so precious these days? The interesting point here is that most people do not appreciate the difference between <u>just getting by</u> and <u>really being and feeling healthy</u>. You see being <u>not</u> sick is <u>not</u> the same as being well and in truth most people are just getting by. What so many people are <u>not</u> doing is enjoying Dynamic Health – they are <u>not</u> looking good and healthy, and/or they're <u>not</u> feeling as well as they could, and/or they're <u>not</u> performing to their reasonable best potential in terms of energy and aches and pains for example, and/or they're running an unnecessarily high risk of developing a disease, even though they may not appreciate that, and their chances of going out like a light-bulb in their 90s, still with all their faculties is, to say the least, <u>slim</u>. But it doesn't have to be that way if we are prepared, in a small way each day, to be proactive and take charge of our health!

On the other hand, I am beginning to meet more and more people who are enjoying Dynamic Health. They often tell me that at the age of say 60, they feel as well as they did aged 30, with less aches and pains and even more energy, but perhaps not as strong and as flexible.

I probably wouldn't have written this book if the level of scientific, medical and clinical knowledge across the world hadn't increased rapidly in the last decade resulting in there now being extremely effective and simple things we can do on a daily basis to enjoy Dynamic Health that were unknown twenty years ago. You will be interested to read at the end of this book about a recent highly significant scientific development, based on Nobel Prize winning physics, which provides the ability to measure the level of antioxidant nutrients in your own body in "real time" in a convenient non-invasive way. This provides you with the ability to measure a very important biomarker of your health – to measure the benefits you are obtaining from your food and supplements. This ability to measure will revolutionise people's ability to manage their health.

I therefore decided that I really had to spread the word! All this new exciting scientifically proven knowledge enables us to become proactive in our lifestyle and nutrition choices on a daily basis, which can help us achieve Dynamic Health. By taking charge in simple ways we can enjoy Dynamic Health for the rest of our lives, which many of us may not have appreciated is now well within our grasp. However, I must make one point very clear;

there are no guarantees of staying in good health and keeping away from disease. On the other hand, it is now possible to move the probabilities substantially in our favour! And remember, the fact that we can measure the benefits of the supplements we are taking, totally changes the world of nutritional supplements. You no longer have to assume or guess whether you're benefiting from the supplement you are taking. You can now have the benefits measured in your body as conclusive proof.

With this safe, reliable and convenient method of measuring antioxidants, we'll begin to see more advances in supplement development and antioxidant research. We'll begin to see a shift from drugs to natural protective measures.

You may have had nagging doubts about whether you and your family will stay fit and healthy for the rest of your lives. You may have become concerned about a particular health issue of a member of your family or yourself. Or you may have raised some queries about your health with the person who pointed you in the direction of this book.

Whatever the reason for your coming across this book, I hope you find it helpful in your Search for Dynamic Health. I advise you to take the information in this book seriously. It can change your life – and the lives of those you love – for the better. Go and get your number measured and then do something to raise it!

INTRODUCTION

From the early 90s man's knowledge of the benefits of beneficial nutrition for promoting human health, has accelerated dramatically! It is hoped that this book will give you some useful basic knowledge on human nutrition and enlighten you on the proven health benefits that can be derived from supplementing your diet, as long as the supplements are of proven quality.

It is assumed from your expression of interest through reading this book that you <u>are</u> interested in your health? But are you prepared to be <u>proactive</u> and <u>invest </u>in your health? Ralph Waldo Emerson once said, *"The first wealth in life is health!"* It doesn't matter how much money you've got; without your health, you have nothing! And this applies to everyone. As a leading vascular surgeon once said, *"Everybody, whether they are an ambassador or a janitor, asks the same questions when they are lying on my operating table with tubes in them!"*

When we talk about and even when we think about enjoying good health, whatever our life's dream is, we need to think of our health before we think of anything else. Think about it – without your health, without a healthy mental state, without abundant energy levels, where would you be? Even if you had all the money, all the capital gains and all the financial security in the world, where would you be without your health? Nowhere!

Here's why! According to a variety of public health surveys, it's clear that the worldwide population in developed countries eats too much, exercises too little and suffers from a growing list of chronic health ailments. This situation is probably no secret to anyone reading this book – in fact it may be quite obvious to you! Look around you! Not only are most adults getting fatter, but our children are doped up on Ritalin, and our parents are battling chronic diseases with prescription medications, as well as suffering the side effects of those powerful drugs.

Among the top 10 best selling prescription drugs, 3 are for treating depression and anxiety, 3 are for lowering cholesterol, 2 are for fighting ulcers, and 2 are painkillers. The interesting thing about these drugs is <u>not</u> the fact that they account for over US$30Billion in annual sales, it is that they all target conditions that are both treatable and preventable with diet and exercise.

Unless you are reading this book as a drug company sales rep or an employee of one of those multinational pharmaceutical companies, it probably makes a lot of sense to you that investing in your <u>own</u> health and wellness will generate long term returns compared to spending your hard earned income on treating the <u>symptoms</u> of a poor lifestyle, let alone exposing yourself to the risks and uncertainties of a Government run Health Service.

In the experience of several highly respected nutritional scientists, who've talked to thousands of successful professionals about their diet and exercise habits over the last six years or so, they can't even count the number of those people who, after having accumulated substantial wealth, have realised that they have done it at the expense of both their mental and physical health. In fact it's a sure bet that it's no consolation to any of those successful men and women that they can now afford the finest room at the convalescent home or the nicest bed in the hospital! In other words, while those captains of industry were out conquering the world, their poor lifestyle habits were conquering themselves!

But there is hope! The good news is that those scientists have yet to meet a single person who has failed to benefit from supplementing their diet and simple alterations to their diet and lifestyle   choices.

THE CHALLENGE

Most modern medicine practices are based on a theory developed by Louis Pasteur. Among his many discoveries and researches, Pasteur is perhaps best known for his germ theory. Pasteur discovered tiny microbes that are present in our environment and our bodies. According to Pasteur's theory, the body is a sterile machine, but when microbes are introduced to that sterile environment, disease results. Pasteur also theorised that certain microbes are responsible for certain diseases. According to the theory, in order to bring the patient back to health, the microbes must be removed. Through employing antibiotics and various chemicals, these illness-causing microbes can be eliminated. In short, no microbes means no illness. Health is defined as the absence of any germ that might cause disease.

This theory tends to divide the body into several different systems. Under the germ theory, it is thought that germs only attack certain parts of the body – certain germs only involve the digestive system, or the respiratory system or any other parts of the body. Therefore, each body system can be treated separately to alleviate illness.

By removing germs from the infected body system, health can be restored. Of course, this theory assumes the rest of the body is healthy. The goal of this treatment is to ensure that each body system is in proper working order, meaning no microbes are present. If each body part is working correctly, then the whole will also be healthy. The very divisions of medicine illustrate the prevalence of the germ theory – doctors specialise in the various different body systems from cardiologists to gastroenterologists.

One of Pasteur's contemporaries had a different idea. The famous physiologist Claude Bernard viewed the body as a whole and emphasised the importance of the internal environment. Bernard taught that microbes could not cause disease unless the body was unbalanced. This natural imbalance, according to Bernard, is conducive to the illnesses caused by microbes. If the body is in balance, then whether microbes are present or not would not matter. A balanced body is able to fight the effects of microbes. Many of these disease-causing microbes are already present in our bodies – in fact many are necessary to perform body functions. Disease results from an imbalance that weakens the body, making it susceptible to the influence of these microbes.

This idea was supported further by the work of Royal R. Rife, the famous microscopist of the 1930s. Rife found that by altering the environment he could make harmless bacteria become toxic. More importantly, Rife found the opposite to be true. By returning the environment to a balanced state, potentially deadly microbes could be returned to a harmless state.

There are, of course, some microbes that are harmful whether the body is balanced or not, like the TB bacteria and the AIDS virus. However, even in these cases the severity of the illness is inversely proportional to the state of the body's internal environment and defence mechanism.

A poorly balanced body results in decreased ability to fight against microbes. In fact, that very imbalance can help the microbes increase. Therefore, overall health is maintained by balancing activity and rest, heat and cold, fat and lean and so forth. Any extreme will result in an imbalance. There are many stressors that can cause your body to slip into imbalance. One of those stressors that can be easily reversed is proper nutrition.

Today's foods are decidedly lacking in the nutrients we need. Although today's foods look and taste good, they do not provide our bodies with the nutrients needed to promote a healthy balance. For many of us, that means we need to take supplements to fill in the gaps caused by our diets.

Modern medicine is slowly moving towards protecting this internal balance. More and more physicians work with their patients to establish proper eating and health habits. Interestingly enough, even Pasteur agreed with Bernard on his deathbed, stating that the environment was everything.

So traditional medicine tells us that germs cause most diseases, and in order to get well we must kill those germs. To achieve that goal the medical profession employs drugs, antibiotics, chemotherapy, radiation, and even surgery.

On the other hand, in recent years there has been a shift in the disease paradigm in that many health professionals and respected medical organisations now accept that disease results from an imbalance in the body. This chaos and disorder in the body is brought on by nutritional imbalance or "intoxication". In order to re-establish health, one needs to balance the body by working with it, not against it!

Any protocol for healing in the human body must be based on a foundation of solid nutrition and diet, which leads to a "balanced body". Proper digestion and a properly functioning immune system are necessary to combat not only foreign bacteria and other pathogens but also the internal damage caused by free oxidizing radical molecules every day. The <u>key</u> to healing the body is <u>balance and antioxidation</u>.

What has been discovered over the last ten years or so is that the common culprits in many diseases are "reactive oxygen species", often called "free radicals". These free radical bad guys, the results of the oxidative process, wreak havoc on the body, creating an imbalance where disease and illness can thrive. However, it has also been discovered that providing our bodies with proper nutrition and supplementation can drastically reduce the number of free radicals and the damage they create to our bodies.

Equally important to achieving balance and antioxidation is that toxins must be eliminated from the body. Detoxification is an essential aspect of the body's healing process. Just as free radicals and toxins can be introduced into the body, they can also be removed, promoting a healthy balance.

What we are basically seeing with the "captains of industry", mentioned earlier, as well as most of the rest of the population, is a "rusting and rotting" effect caused by the very foods we eat. It is much like a car. No one can deny that the salt thrown down on icy roads is a necessary part of winter driving, however, that very salt promotes rust and damage to cars. Many of the foods that we eat have similar effects on our bodies. Too much salt, sugar, caffeine, meat, fats, and other substances are detrimental to the balance that we seek to maintain. Yet, how many of us are prepared to give up or at least moderate intake of those things?

There is an old joke about a man who goes to the doctor and is told to give up everything he enjoys. When the doctor tells him to stop smoking, drinking, staying up late, and eating rich foods, the man asks, "Doctor, if I do these things, will you guarantee that I will live to be 100 years old?" The doctor looks the man in the eyes and says, "No, but I guarantee that it will seem like 100 years!"

Living a full and healthy life certainly does not mean giving up everything that makes life worth living. But it does require that we make a commitment to wellness, i.e. being healthy, based on responsible decisions about nutrition and lifestyle. By seeking balance through nutrition and supplementation – geared to eliminating the damage caused by free radicals –

you will find that life can be so much more fulfilling!

It is hoped that this book will help you discover and establish solid principles, which will enable you and your family to not only stay healthy, but to become even more healthy – or, if you are suffering health challenges, how to improve your health. Your understanding of the principles of antioxidation and the use of antioxidants through diet and supplements will go a very long way towards assuring you of Dynamic Health for the rest of your life.

THE SEARCH FOR DYNAMIC HEALTH

BACKGROUND

Up to the mid 90's, generally speaking, medical teaching said that to be healthy, all you need to be is a healthy person eating a healthy and balanced diet, not smoking, and taking exercise. That is still the belief of many people at the start of the 21st Century, and it is of course correct to say that you should not smoke and you should take regular exercise. However, many people do not yet appreciate that it is now a proven fact that we can no longer obtain everything we need from our food, not even from a well-balanced diet, if we want to enjoy Dynamic Health. "The well-balanced diet is no longer an option if we want our health to be anything above adequate!"

So what is Dynamic Health? Dynamic Health allows you to perform at 80 as if you were 50; it enables you to look good, feel good, perform better, keep away from disease, and die young as late as possible! Due to substantial advances in scientific knowledge since the mid-90s, this is now something that <u>can</u> be achieved through a proactive approach to life. You can feel better at 60 than you did aged 30.

Jeffrey Blumberg, Assistant Director of the Center on Ageing at Tufts University, USA said – *"We think of health negatively, as an absence of sickness. Being <u>not</u> sick is <u>not</u> the same as being well."*

Ken Dychtwald, a top demographic expert in the USA, said – *"A lifetime of disregard for personal health usually leads, not to a death sentence, but to chronic disease. What you do in your 30's and 40's can, in many cases, trap you in a diseased body in your 50's and 60's."*

Ashley Montagu, the Anthropologist stated, *"The goal of life is to die young as late as possible."*

In industrialised nations, 85% of the population over 65 is chronically ill. The U.S. spends more than $26Billion annually on those people who have lost their independence because of degenerative diseases. Much of this illness and expense can be avoided by maintaining our bodies in a healthy balanced state.

An American Dietetic Association survey in 1997 showed that 35% of people believed that they needed to take vitamin supplements for good health. What is more interesting is that just 2 years earlier, only 25% believed they should supplement their diet. It took only 2 years for another 10% of the population to believe they should supplement their diets!

Frost and Sullivan, a market research firm, carried out a survey at the same time, which concluded that the substantial increase in the US Vitamin and Supplement market to around $5.8 Billion a year was due to three market drivers:

1. Dissatisfaction with conventional medicines,

2. Social trends towards good health, self care, and health maintenance
3. Population growth.

Frost and Sullivan said, *"It is abundantly clear that people in the Western world are becoming aware that they need "to take charge" of their health."* Indeed, in 1999 the World Trade Organisation forecast that over the 10 years to 2010 the Global Nutritional Supplement Market would increase 5-fold from $62 Billion to over $300 Billion!

At no other time in our history has the public interest in self-care and the use of natural health remedies been so widespread. More than 50% of the adult population of the US, Japan, and most of Europe are now consuming a dietary supplement on a regular basis. From these statistics it's clear that the acceptance of using dietary supplements to promote health and reduce disease is here to stay.

The vast majority of people in industrialised countries, including as much as 80% of the population of the US, Japan, and Europe feel that they just don't consume adequate levels of vitamins and minerals from their diets. National Nutrition Surveys in those parts of the world support this perception. For example, statistics from the US Department of Agriculture, the USDA, indicate that less than 1% of American adults regularly take in 5 servings of fruits and vegetables every day and the American Cancer Society recommends people should eat 5 to 10 servings of fruit and vegetables a day! More than 70% of the US population fails to achieve even the low RDA levels for many vitamins and nutrients.

People are now appreciating that the overloaded medical profession, which has to cope with crisis after crisis, because of an ageing population, is probably not the place to go to learn how to achieve Dynamic Health. Also, most doctors have received very little training on nutrition. Some would openly admit that they received only 5 hours of instruction on nutrition out of a total of 5,000 hours, and they were the lucky ones! Many doctors will tell you that, when they were students, they were taught that unless there were symptoms of vitamin deficiency, the only people that would gain by taking vitamin supplements were the manufacturers! This understandable "ingrained attitude" is compounded further by sensational announcements about vitamins etc. in the Press, followed a few weeks later by similarly sensational headlines with completely opposing views! Attitudes are changing fast in the Medical profession because of the scientific and clinical evidence, which is becoming available, but even so, their area of responsibility inevitably remains primarily at the crisis end of health rather than prevention. <u>Prevention, not cure, is the answer!</u>

There is now an emerging market for Nutraceuticals, which are Nutritional Supplements made using pharmaceutical methodologies, i.e. they are made to the lowest marker molecule. Increasingly people are viewing drugs as negative because of the clinical evidence that many drugs produce adverse side effects including serious nutrient depletion. You will be interested to know that the book, "Drug-Induced Nutrient Depletion Handbook" from Lexi-Comp's Clinical Reference Library runs to nearly 500 pages! People are therefore looking for natural alternatives and increasingly want scientific proof that such natural nutritional supplements are safe and work.

Unfortunately, "natural" products are not necessarily safe and do not always provide the benefits indicated. Independent analyses have shown in several cases that the product offered had not been taken from the correct part of the plant resulting in the product not including the scientifically proven appropriate active ingredient. In extreme cases, there was none of the particular plant, described on the label, in the bottle <u>and some were even spiked with synthetic drugs!</u>

It should therefore be no surprise that nearly all nutritional/dietary supplements in the health food shops and pharmacies are <u>not</u> pharmaceutical grade and are not clinically proven on humans to be safe or efficacious, i.e. deliver on their promise. A typical example of this is a survey that was carried out on all the Ginseng products on the US market. It showed that over 85% of the Ginseng products on the shelves had fungicide levels in the bottles that were above the US legal limits! It is therefore important to ensure that any company's products that you are thinking of buying are supported by peer-reviewed scientific studies, preferably randomised double blind placebo controlled clinical studies on humans, and are subjected to a rigorous quality control process, which together prove that the products are safe and work.

Recent scientific research is throwing up whole new areas of knowledge, concerning human nutrition, much of which comes from the plant kingdom. In particular, Phytochemicals are beginning to revolutionise human nutrition. Newsweek, USA published a headline article on Phytonutrients on 25th April 1994. It said *"Just a few years ago, scientists didn't know phytochemicals existed. But today they are the new frontier in cancer-prevention research."*

It is a salutary thought that the Chinese, who are reputedly the oldest civilisation in the world, have been using herbs and plants for centuries – for what? In the Orient, to maintain your health, you pay the doctor to keep you in good health, not just to treat you when you are ill! The emphasis is on prevention not cure. In the Western world the emphasis is the other way round, i.e. on cure or crisis. You have to be ill first before you go to the doctor! It should therefore be no surprise that the population in the Western world is moving fast towards Oriental principles. It is now scientifically proven that there are over 300 plant chemicals (phytonutrients), which can provide substantial and indeed critical health benefits to the human body. This Phytochemical breakthrough in the 90s is considered by many to be as significant to human health as the creation of Antibiotics!

Phytochemicals or phytonutrients come from whole fruits and vegetables. The American

Cancer Society recommends that the daily intake of fruits and vegetables for every adult should be at least 5 and preferably 10 servings or more a day. However, the average American diet, which is similar to other Western diets, is well short of that, including barely 3 servings of fruits and vegetables daily and one of those is "French Fries"! So, on average, we are getting only 25% or less of the ideal intake of phytochemicals that we need day-by-day, i.e. we are 75% or more short! That will inevitably take its toll on our health unless we correct that imbalance!

This rapidly increasing awareness amongst the population, that there <u>are</u> nutritional solutions to achieving "Dynamic Health", is being fuelled by the "Ageing of the Baby Boomers", who are searching for any way possible to hold onto their youth. What is "Dynamic Health"? People enjoying Dynamic Health would "look good, feel good, perform better, keep away from disease, and die young as late as possible!"

The challenge is that the environment is becoming more toxic and farming and food processing methods as well as storage and transport are delivering much lower levels of nutrients in our food than a century ago. In addition our lifestyle has become more sedentary which is putting us out of step with our evolution.

The cells in our bodies, other than our brain cells, replicate themselves at least every 7 years but in many cases every few months. Some regenerate in just a few days and even in hours!

We can even create new brain cells to a limited degree! The question therefore is – "Where does all the material come from to support our bodies in this cell replicating and life maintaining process?" It can only come from the material we ingest, i.e. our food.

There is a great saying in the computer industry, "Garbage in – garbage out!" The human body is as much a process as a computer system or any other system for that matter; it needs to be kept in balance. Garbage food, which lacks the many nutrients that our bodies need, as well as including undesirable constituents, will result in garbage, i.e. toxins being ingested into our blood stream. This "garbage" has to be screened out by our liver or kidneys and our immune system so that it won't damage the cells of our bodies. In time that damage, if left unchecked, could lead to organ failure in the body. In any case, where are all the essential nutrients to enable the DNA in our cells to recreate themselves as perfectly as possible in the garbage? Answer, probably nowhere! So our body cells have to make do with inferior "fuel", which damages them and makes it difficult for them to replicate themselves correctly, resulting in the death of some of those cells. We are already intensifying the ageing process, which is the accumulating loss of body cells! Also, in that scenario, we are risking one or more of the organs in our bodies becoming damaged, due to taking in toxic food/fuel that creates free radical oxidative damage, which our bodies are continuously exposed to and which is implicated in around 75% of all diseases.

Deprived of the nutrients they need, our bodies become out of balance and slowly cave in to the accumulation of damage, mainly from reactive oxygen species, throughout our lives. If, however, we provide our bodies regularly with the quality nutrients they need and can use, then our lives, and the quality of our lives, will be enhanced, in many cases immeasurably.

FREE RADICALS CREATE OXIDATIVE DAMAGE

Your body needs oxygen to produce energy. Think of it as a fire. By adding wood to a flame, you can create heat. Without oxygen, your body cannot process the fuel you give it to provide you with energy. Oxygen quite literally helps you "burn calories".

Energy is produced in your body through a process called "oxidation". Basically, your body employs paired electrons from oxygen to produce energy. This process also creates by-products – like smoke and ash from fires, which are called reactive oxygen species. These reactive oxygen species are the dangerous free radicals that cause oxidative damage to your cells.

Most people know that atoms are the basic particle of a chemical element. These atoms are further broken down into electrons travelling around neutrons in orbitals. Electrons like to be found in pairs – the orbitals that they travel in can hold a maximum of two electrons. When an atom has an odd number of electrons, it becomes very reactive – searching out another electron to fill out its orbitals. These atoms or molecules that lack an electron are called "reactive oxygen species" or free radicals.

There are 12 different types of Reactive Oxygen Species or Free Radicals. Oxidative damage is the common denominator in the process of ageing and its associated diseases. Each cell in our body, on average, is subjected to 73,000 free radical attacks on its DNA every day! Free

Radical damage comes from changes in environmental, dietary, physical, and psychological situations, which produce in the body an abundance of toxic oxygen-free radicals, which attack DNA and damage cell membranes. Our defence against this constant attack has always been antioxidants, mainly in fruits and vegetables, which we have ingested on a hit and miss basis, dependent on the food we happen to eat!

Unstable Toxic Oxygen-Free Radicals can be stabilised by Antioxidants. In simple terms, Free Radicals are unstable toxic molecules, which have an unpaired electron in their orbiting ring. Antioxidants are molecules, which have extra electrons in their orbiting ring, one of which they can give up to a free radical to stabilise it, without themselves turning into a free radical. This stops the damaging chain reaction in our bodies, which leads to premature ageing and is implicated in around 75% of all diseases.

Oxygen is the basis of all plant and animal life. It is our most important nutrient, needed by every cell every second of every day. Without it we cannot release the energy from food, which drives all our body processes. But oxygen is chemically reactive and highly dangerous! In normal biochemical reactions oxygen can become unstable and capable of "oxidising" neighbouring molecules. This can lead to cellular damage, which triggers cancer, inflammation, arterial damage, and ageing. Known as reactive oxygen species, this bodily equivalent of nuclear waste must be disarmed to remove the danger.

This process of oxidation can be easily illustrated by cutting an apple in half. If you leave one half of the apple exposed long enough to the air, you'll see a brown mush forming on it. This is due to the healthy cells of the apple reacting with the free radicals present in our environment. Slowly the healthy cells of the apple are broken down into the less appealing mush. Rust on your car is yet another example of damage from oxidation. If however you dip the other half of the apple in lemon juice, which includes the antioxidant vitamin C, you will see that the cut surface of that half does not go brown anywhere near so quickly. This is because the vitamin C in the lemon juice is protecting the apple by giving up its extra electrons to the environment rather than the apple losing an electron to the environment. This is exactly how antioxidants protect the cells in your body.

Examining red blood cells under a microscope can provide another example of cellular damage. If you compare red blood cells of a non-smoker with those of a smoker, you will see the comparative damage to the red blood cells of the smoker, by their significant jagged edges, compared to the red blood cells of the non-smoker with their normal smooth edges. The damaged red blood cells of the smoker will not be as effective at carrying oxygen as undamaged cells.

Free radicals come from pollution and are made in all combustion processes including smoking, the burning of petrol to create exhaust fumes, radiation, frying or barbecuing food. Our normal body metabolic processes including the digestion of food and handling of stress also produce them. Indeed, around 3% of all the oxygen we breathe in is left over as waste from our metabolic processes and is known as Superoxide, which is the most common free radical our bodies have to deal with.

In its natural everyday functions including the handling of stress, your body will produce literally millions of free radicals. When you throw into the melee the free radicals that are present throughout our environment from pollution, toxins, radiation, and poor foods, you soon have an overwhelmed defence system – one that cannot keep up with all the damage. This results in a serious imbalance occurring in the body, which lays it open to microbe invasion and accelerated ageing.

Free Radicals do not seem overly dangerous until you consider where they are causing their damage. If a free radical steals an electron from an atom making up the DNA of a cell, Cancer can result. Or if the free radical damages a cell wall, it can lead to the premature death of that cell. There are limitless possibilities of damage that a free radical can cause simply by "borrowing an electron", which cuts a link in the molecular structure at random and sets off a chain reaction of molecular destabilisation throughout the body.

Free radicals can cause damage to virtually all parts of the body. Most notably, free radicals can damage your DNA. DNA acts as the blueprint to your cells. When it is damaged, vital functions necessary for the cell's continued health can be shut down or, in the case of Cancer, can be thrown out of balance. Proteins can also be damaged by free radicals. Your body uses proteins to make many of the cells, enzymes, and hormones that it needs. When the proteins are damaged, production of these components is slowed, creating another imbalance.

Free radicals can also make proteins fuse together, causing them not to function properly. The most noticeable area where this happens is in the skin because the ultra-violet rays in sunlight cause skin protein molecules, or collagen, to fuse together, giving the skin a "leathery" appearance.

The most frequent damage caused by free radicals involves fatty compounds called "lipids". This damage to lipids is called "lipid peroxidation". We are all familiar with lipid peroxidation. Whenever we speak of something going "rancid", we are actually talking about lipid peroxidation. Fats react quickly to free radicals, which is one reason why people who are fat, and especially those who are obese, could be more at risk of developing Cancer than people with a normal body mass index and an acceptable body fat percentage.

However, lipids are not just stored body fat; they are also used in hormone-like substances and in cell membranes. If cell membranes are damaged by free radicals then the cell is no longer able to import needed nutrients and oxygen and to export waste products and carbon dioxide. This can result in the death of cells, the critical factor in ageing. Ageing is fundamentally the loss of body cells, which, if not kept in check, can accelerate over time.

DNA and cell membranes are not the only victims of free radicals at the cellular level. Free radicals can also damage lysosomes. Lysosomes are like storage sacks filled with enzymes that break down foreign materials and pathogens, such as bacteria, viruses and fungi. If the membranes that hold these enzymes are damaged, allowing them to leak, then the enzymes will actually start breaking down other cellular components in the body.

FREE RADICALS AND AGEING

Free Radicals and Ageing are strongly linked. Risks of contracting more than 80 "age-related" diseases can be alleviated by antioxidants that neutralise oxidant particles. Many of the diseases that doctors attribute to time are actually directly related to the accumulation of free radical damage in the cells of the body, and this accumulation of damage can be changed. Ageing might best be described as the slow and continuous loss of body cells, i.e. a reduction of the number of cells in the body.

Many of the physical effects we call "Ageing" are the result of the "rusting and rotting" effect on our bodies of the continuous daily damage to the cells in our bodies caused by reactive oxygen species. Ageing is not the "wearing out" of body parts. Rather, ageing is the accumulation of damage to individual cells all over the body. The damage from this normal oxidative process in living cells results in cell degeneration and death, which in turn lead to the problems that we associate with ageing.

It's very similar to your car. By practicing regular maintenance habits, your car's life can be lengthened. But imagine what would happen if you only used the lowest grade fuel available, never changed the oil, never took your car to the mechanic, and never washed your car. Your car's lifespan would be considerably reduced – even if you were never involved in an accident. By keeping your car properly maintained and protected by high quality liquids and parts, your car can run much more efficiently and longer.

Ageing is not the measurement of time, but rather it is a measurement of cells. As we maintain a properly balanced environment for our bodies, cells are able to continue their work uninterrupted. But when faced with imbalance, our bodies and all their constituent parts and organs begin to lose cells until the much-needed reserve levels of cells are depleted, and we succumb to the accumulated damage, often resulting in organ failure or the onset of life-threatening and/or degenerative diseases, which in some cases can occur relatively early in life.

FREE RADICALS AND DISEASES

Not only can Free Radicals throw our bodies into an unbalanced state, making them more receptive to microbes and other pathogens, they can also contribute to many diseases.

According to a list that was published in "The Annals of Internal Medicine" (1987, 107:527), **Free Radicals can promote:**

> Ageing – premature ageing and immune system deficiency
> Cancers
> Cardiovascular disease
> Autoimmune disease
> Rheumatoid arthritis
> Amyloid degenerative diseases
> Radiation injury
> Cataracts
> Porphyria (psychological and physical disorders due to porphyrin build up in body)
> Retinopathy
> Parkinson's disease

According to Chapter 13 in "The Optimum Nutrition Bible" by Patrick Holford (Founder of the Institute of Optimum Nutrition), published in 1997 in London –

Probable Antioxidant Deficiency Diseases are as follows:

> Alzheimer's disease
> Cancer * (see next paragraph)
> Cardiovascular disease * (see next paragraph)

Cataracts
Diabetes * (see next paragraph)
Hypertension
Infertility
Macular degeneration of the eye (see next
    paragraph)
Mental illness
Periodontal disease
Respiratory tract infections
Rheumatoid arthritis

* "Over 75% of people in the Western World will die or experience severe disabilities from these 3 diseases, Cancer, Cardiovascular disease, and Diabetes alone, and oxidative free radical damage is implicated in all these diseases! The only answer to this situation is to have, every minute of every hour of every day of every year, a powerful mix of antioxidants circulating in the blood to continually scavenge for free radicals!"

As mentioned earlier, one aspect of enjoying "Dynamic Health" is "keeping away from disease". Disease is the antithesis of good health, so in order to talk about health constructively it is necessary to consider diseases, which could take away our health, let alone Dynamic Health. So let's talk briefly about the 3 pervasive diseases mentioned above plus Macular Degeneration of the retina of the eye, which leads to impaired vision and often blindness in so many people after the age of 65. Remember, the following four diseases account for nearly 80% of all deaths and severe disabilities:

CANCER. In the United States, there are approximately 4 million people who have Cancer and probably more than double that in Europe. Of these, around a third will eventually die from the disease. Although there are many variants of Cancer, there is a common thread running through them all – free radicals contribute in a major way to their development.

Cancer is the uncontrolled growth of body cells. Through damage to the DNA, a cell begins to replicate itself at an abnormal rate. Eventually, this uncontrolled growth forms tumours and can lead to other problems such as individual organs in the body failing. These cells, especially when they are invasive, may also "migrate" or metastasise to other parts of the body, where they can create secondary cancers or metastases.

Your body has natural defences against such problems. However, in today's world, with many different carcinogenic substances in our environment, our defences are swamped, especially when they're not getting the right kind of defensive supplies from the food we eat. Add to that the damage that our bodies must repair just from daily living, and soon our bodies just can't keep up!

As has been said earlier, one of the ways that DNA can be damaged is by free radicals. If a free radical "borrows" an electron from a strain of DNA, the cell can become cancerous. Antioxidants act against this "borrowing" process by providing free radicals with the electrons they need.

Antioxidants also work to help the liver function properly. When functioning at full capacity, the liver will eliminate 99% of the toxins in the body. But when damaged and under-supplied, the liver's effectiveness drops. With the help of antioxidants, the liver can filter out the toxins that our body suffers from.

Finally, antioxidants help boost the immune system, the system responsible for finding and eliminating cancerous and abnormal cells as well as pathogens – bacteria, viruses, and fungi. Clearly the most sensible policy towards such a pervasive disease as Cancer is "prevention". The key antioxidants that are clinically proven in tens of thousands of clinical studies across the world to have the ability to provide protection against Cancer are Vitamins E and C, Selenium, Alpha-Lipoic Acid, Beta-Carotene, the Bioflavonoids, including the Anthocyanins, especially Grape Seed Extract, and Green Tea, especially its Catechins, the most powerful of which is Epigallocatechin Gallate (EGCg). These are expanded on later in this book under "The First Pillar of Health" – Antioxidants and "The Second Pillar of Health" – Phytonutrients.

CARDIOVASCULAR DISEASE. Around half the deaths in the United States and Europe are attributed to cardiovascular disease. Heart attack and stroke are the first and third leading causes of death. Arteriosclerosis, the major cause of cardiovascular disease, is entirely preventable!

There are many causes of cardiovascular disease but arteriosclerosis is the main contributor to the problem. Commonly thought of as "hardening" of the arteries, arteriosclerosis is actually more like "clogging" of the arteries. The inside of the arteries becomes filled with a build-up of plaque containing cholesterol, fats, and other junk. This build-up closes off the arteries, decreasing the amount of blood flowing through the blood vessels while increasing blood pressure. Imagine your garden hose. When you block off part of the end of the hose less water comes out but at an increased pressure. This same situation is happening in your arteries! Though less blood can pass through them, your heart still pumps the same amount, increasing the pressure.

Additionally, pieces of plaque can break off from arterial walls. When these pieces of plaque flow to the brain, they can cause blockages in the millions of blood vessels there, leading to stroke. Arteriosclerosis starts with damage to the lining of the arteries, known as the endothelium. When the endothelium is damaged, small lesions or cuts are formed. This damage is caused by free radicals. As they attack the cells that make up the endothelium, they create these small cuts. In fact, if you place a healthy blood vessel in a dish of hydrogen peroxide, which produces oxidative damage, you can watch the endothelium dissolve!

These small lesions provide excellent areas for fats, high levels of the amino acid, homocysteine, and other junk to attach to the artery wall. When the endothelium is damaged, the immune system sends out cells for damage control. The result is big, puffy cells that can easily snag on the lesions in the endothelium. These cells are known as "foam cells". LDL cholesterol (bad) is also very susceptible to the same free radicals that damage the endothelium. When LDL is oxidised, it becomes sticky, clinging to the artery walls and blocking them. HDL cholesterol (good) doesn't have the same problem and can even help to clean up some of the problems caused by damaged LDLs. But when foam cells combine with oxidised LDL cholesterol, you have a serious situation on your hands because your body can't keep up!

The true problem lies in the build-up of these complications. Allowing this process to continue only adds layers to the plaque that is forming in the arteries. As the plaque builds up, it reduces the blood vessel's ability to push the blood along. Normally, blood vessels have their own contracting motion, which helps blood flow. However, when a layer of plaque has built up, these contractions are nullified. Imagine being massaged through a 4-inch foam pad on your back. It kind of defeats the purpose! When your blood vessels can't help, the workload falls back on your heart.

Now imagine the result of all these complications added together. Less blood is flowing through your body but at an increased pressure. Your blood vessels can't help move the blood along, which makes the heart have to push harder. Because there is less blood reaching your body, signals are sent to your heart to increase the amount of blood being pumped, causing your heart to race all the time. This is a less than optimal situation for your cardiovascular health! The sad aspect of all this is that you may not even notice this is happening until it is too late because an artery can become 90% blocked without the person being restricted in his activities! Cardiovascular disease is known as the "silent killer" because the first symptom that is noticed is often a fatal heart attack.

With early detection, a change in lifestyle habits and diet can help to reverse the damage. If not, surgery is another option but it carries its own set of risks and problems. The best course of action is early prevention.

How do we go about preventing cardiovascular disease? One of the easiest and best changes to make is physical activity. As a society, we are becoming increasingly sedentary – we are getting out of step with our evolution! By increasing our physical activity, we increase our cardiovascular health. Both the American Heart Association and the American Council on Exercise recommend an hour of light exercise 3 to 5 times a week.

Another major prevention step that you can take to prevent cardiovascular disease is to prevent damage to your endothelium, the lining to your arteries. This means stopping oxidative damage in its tracks. And how do you do this? Through antioxidants, plus, where appropriate, reducing cholesterol and homocysteine levels in the blood!

Low antioxidant levels have consistently been associated with increased risk of cardiovascular disease. Oxidative damage to blood vessel walls as well as damage to LDL cholesterol is the primary cause of arteriosclerosis. A broad spectrum or network of antioxidants is called for in protecting these fatty tissues and cells. The most important of these antioxidants are Vitamins E and C, Selenium, and the Carotenoids, Beta-carotene, Lycopene, and Lutein.

Vitamin E may be the single most important antioxidant when it comes to cardiovascular health. LDL readily incorporates it and vitamin E protects it from free radical damage. Vitamin E also helps reduce LDL cholesterol levels, raise good HDL cholesterol levels, inhibit platelet aggregation, and break down excess fibrogen.

Vitamin C is important as an antioxidant for two reasons. First, it acts to prevent oxidative damage caused by free radicals. Secondly, and perhaps more importantly, vitamin C helps other antioxidants to do their jobs and helps to regenerate them. Vitamin C actually helps recycle vitamin E, requiring you to consume less. Vitamin C lowers cholesterol levels and blood pressure as well.

The Carotenoids – e.g. Beta Carotene, Lycopene, and Lutein provide essential additional support for cardiovascular health. (For benefits see "The First Pillar of Health" – Antioxidants later in this book.)

DIABETES. Diabetes is manifested by elevations of fasting sugar levels. A chronic disorder of carbohydrate, fat, and protein metabolism, diabetes places its sufferers at increased risk of heart disease, cerebral vascular stroke, kidney disease, eye disease and diabetic neuropathy, or impairment of the peripheral nerve function.

In diabetics, either the pancreas does not produce enough insulin, or the cells in the body have grown resistant to the take-up of insulin. In either case, blood sugar cannot enter the cells (insulin resistance), which can cause serious health problems.

There are two types of diabetes: Type 1 and Type 2. Type 1 diabetes is an insulin-dependent diabetes occurring mostly before and during adolescence. Type 2, or non-insulin dependent diabetes, which up to now has generally occurred after the age of 40 and is often called "Age-related onset Diabetes", is strongly related to obesity. Due to increasing obesity in the young, Type 2 diabetes is concerningly occurring in teenagers and those in their twenties, making the description "Age-related onset Diabetes" sadly less appropriate!

The symptoms, frequent urination, excessive appetite, and excessive thirst, are generally the same for both types of diabetes. Other symptoms include blurring of vision, itching of the skin, fatigue, slow wound healing, and skin infections associated with tingling and numbness of the feet. Diabetics may also have increased facial hair, loss of leg hair, and small yellow bumps on the body.

The exact cause of Type I diabetes is not known, but a current theory is that injury to the pancreas, coupled with some defect in the pancreatic tissue's ability to regenerate itself, produces diabetes. In Type I diabetes, the immune system apparently attacks the pancreas, a condition that is strongly related to free radical damage.

90% of all Diabetics are Type 2, which is again a condition that is strongly related to free radical damage. In Type 2 diabetes, insulin levels are elevated, indicating a loss of cellular sensitivity to insulin. Obesity is a contributory factor in the majority of Type 2 cases, which should be no surprise when one considers the high rates of increase in both those people developing Type 2 diabetes and people becoming obese! Returning to a healthy body weight with an acceptable body mass index and body fat percentage usually results in a restoration of normal blood sugar levels.

The transportation of vitamin C into the body cells is accomplished through insulin. Because of this, diabetics are often deficient in their levels of intracellular vitamin C. This vitamin C deficiency can lead to many of the problems that we have already looked at including vascular disease, elevation of cholesterol, and a significantly depressed immune system, increasing the risk of Cancer.

High doses of vitamin C also reduce the accumulation of Sorbitol in red blood cells. Sorbitol is associated with many of the complications that diabetics suffer from, especially eye and nerve disorders.

Vitamin E increases insulin action. Reducing overall oxidative stress through vitamin E helps reduce the long-term problems that face diabetics. Vitamin E also appears to play a role in preventing diabetes. One study showed that low vitamin E blood levels were associated with a 4 times greater risk of developing diabetes.

Zinc has a powerful protective effect on the pancreas, preventing oxidative damage to the organ. Diabetics typically excrete excessive amounts of zinc (which is the most important mineral needed by the body, and a constituent of over 200 enzymes), so supplementation is needed. Zinc improves insulin levels in both Type 1 and Type 2 diabetics.

MACULAR DEGENERATION.

Macular Degeneration will cause 20% of people over the age of 65 to lose all or part of their vision. Those over the age of 75 face a 37% chance of losing their sight to the same disease.

Macular degeneration is the degradation of the macula, the part of the retina where light focuses after it passes through the lens and the eyeball. The macula can degenerate in two ways. First, due to a lack of pigments that act as filters for harmful light rays, the macula is subjected to free radical damage caused by light radiation. Second, proliferation of capillaries around the macula can cause damage. These capillaries can leak, causing the formation of scar tissue. The scar tissue can cause the retina to detach from its protective covering, or the scar tissue can distort the shape of the retina. Either way, the light is not focussed correctly, and nerve impulses are interfered with, resulting in seriously impaired vision.

The first symptoms of macular degeneration are decreased clarity of vision and distortion of shapes. As the disease progresses light is focussed more on scar tissue, and the central area of vision is decreased until nothing is left.

The primary cause of this disease is lipid peroxidation due to free radical attack. Blood profiles of patients suffering from macular degeneration show low levels of selenium and glutathione but high levels of oxidised glutathione. This means the body uses up all the glutathione available in fighting hydrogen peroxide, and none is left to protect the eyes. Selenium is used by the body to convert oxidised glutathione into useable glutathione. Therefore, low levels of selenium are indicative of free radical damage. In the case of macular degeneration, hydrogen peroxide attacks the capillaries of the eye, which are rich in fatty deposits. This causes leaking and the formation of scar tissue.

The only effective treatment for this condition is to destroy the capillaries with a laser. However, the capillaries can grow back, leaving the patient no better off.

Proper nutrition will not reverse this condition, but it will go a long way towards preventing it. The only way to correct the deficit of useable glutathione is to take more **Selenium**. The body uses selenium to recycle glutathione that has been oxidised. With increased levels of glutathione, the body is better equipped to protect the eyes.

Ginkgo Biloba increases blood flow in capillary networks, relaxes the capillaries, and repairs oxidative damage to capillary walls. By increasing the health of the capillaries, you decrease the chance of developing macular degeneration.

Your mother was partially right – carrots will help your vision. While they may not give you better vision, the Carotenoids in them will help protect your eyes. **Carotenoids**, specifically Lutein and Zeaxanthin, have been associated with a 43% drop in the chance of developing macular degeneration. Both Lutein and Zeaxanthin are concentrated in the retina and help prevent free radical damage there. They also promote the levels of pigments that act as filters for harmful light rays.

Zinc is the most plentiful mineral in the eye. However, the elderly suffer from a drop in their zinc levels, making them more susceptible to macular degeneration. Studies have shown that patients given zinc supplements have a decreased likelihood of developing macular degeneration.

ANTIOXIDANTS

Free Radical Damage can occur anywhere in your body. Your body naturally regulates the process of oxidation. Defences are in place to react with reactive oxygen species, controlling the amount of damage they can cause. However, environmental factors, and even other conditions within our bodies including stress, are increasing the amount of free radicals our bodies have to deal with.

Below is a short list of some of the factors that lead to increased levels of free radicals:

Stress – emotional or physical stress that makes you breathe less and burn energy more. Stress feeds on anaerobic metabolism rather than oxygen, thus creating free radicals.

Ozone – produces Superoxide, a common type of free radical.

Auto exhaust – from your car creates carbon monoxide and other substances that take the place of oxygen as you breathe, creating more free radicals.

Cigarette Smoke – similar to auto exhaust; cigarette smoke, including billions of free radicals from one cigarette, takes the place of oxygen, meaning a smoker and those nearby breathe in vast amounts of free radicals rather than oxygen.

Inflammations – your body creates free radicals as it fights illness.

Radiation – like sunlight, alters molecules turning them into free radicals.

Processed foods – do not provide the nutrients needed to support aerobic metabolism, so your body shifts to anaerobic metabolism to produce energy, which creates free radicals.

Drugs – even drugs that your doctor may prescribe for you change your ability to metabolise oxygen, thus creating free radicals.

Free radicals are present everywhere you go. Whether you are producing them in natural body functions or taking them in from the environment, your body is continually fighting against the ravages of free radicals. But your body has limits – it can only do so much. It is up to you to help your body overcome these ill effects by supplying it continuously with a broad spectrum of antioxidants.

Antioxidants protect the body in 4 ways:

- Antioxidants <u>prevent</u> free radicals from forming.
- Antioxidants <u>intercept</u> free radicals that have already formed.
- Antioxidants <u>build up</u> the body's defences.
- Antioxidants <u>eliminate and replace</u> damaged molecules.

As antibiotics in the last 50 years of the 20th century helped "cure" many infectious diseases, so antioxidants will affect a "cure" and protect against many supposedly incurable diseases in the 21st century and slow the process of ageing dramatically. This is good news, but few of us, including many doctors, have ever heard of this Antioxidant Revolution!

You will no doubt be interested, if not amused, to know that – the word, "Antioxidant" is not included in the 64-page Index to the British Medical Association – "Complete Family Health Guide"! Also, the section on "Vitamin and Mineral Supplements" is only allotted 3 pages out of a total of 1,104! The whole theme of the Guide is, understandably, – "Crisis, Cure and Drugs" – not – "Prevention". Indeed, a more appropriate title might be – "Complete Family Disease Guide". In truth Doctors are in the "Disease" Business not the "Health" Business!

In contrast, America's 8 million copy "Best Seller", the #1 Guide to Natural Health – "Prescription for Nutritional Healing" by Phyllis A. Balch CNC and James F. Balch M.D., runs to 776 pages! You should also know that because pharmaceutical drugs are clinically proven to produce so many side effects, some of which are serious, the "Drug-Induced Nutrient Depletion Handbook" – 1999-2000 runs to as many as 485 pages!

As has been said earlier, the key to good health is to feed the body with quality nutrients in the right quantities to ensure it never runs short of anything, to support its metabolic processes continually and help it keep away from disease and all the complications that can result from the resultant drug therapy prescribed to cure the disease in the first place. As Paul Zane Pilzer, an advisor to two US Presidential Administrations said in his book, The Next

<u>Trillion</u>, *"You should make your medicine your food and your food your medicine."*

This "Preventative Approach" is much less costly than the "Cure Approach", which is like shutting the door after the horse has bolted! Treating disease and all the side effects of complicit prescription drugs, plus coping with the resulting incapacities from those diseases, especially of the elderly, including "early-onset" ageing, is incredibly expensive. The United States alone spends around $25 Billion a year caring for the chronically incapacitated – that is a cost of $100 a year for every man, woman and child!

This, of course, only covers the cost angle; it ignores the benefits of the "Preventative Approach" to achieving Dynamic Health, which are that you should "look good, feel good, perform better, keep away from disease, and die young, i.e. with all your faculties functioning, as late as possible! The unique advantage of enjoying Dynamic Health is that you can enjoy those benefits every second of every minute of every hour of every day of every year! Without doubt, the greatest investment you can make is in your health! Remember what Ralph Waldo Emerson said, "The first Wealth in life is Health!"

Dr Lester Packer, PhD., the Father of Antioxidant Theory, based at the University of California at Berkeley says: "There is Overwhelming Evidence that Oxidative Stress (Free Radical Damage) and Disease are Linked". "70% of Americans will die prematurely from diseases caused by or compounded by deficiencies of antioxidants"!

Dr Packer is President of the International Society for Free Radical Research and Vice President of UNESCO's Global Network of Molecular and Cell Biology and is a member of 8 Professional societies. He has published 700 scientific papers and 70 books on every aspect of antioxidants and health, including the standard references *"Vitamin E in Health and Disease"*, *"Vitamin C in Health and Disease"*, *"The Handbook of Natural Antioxidants"* and *"Understanding the Process of Ageing: The Roles of Mitochondria, Free Radicals, and Antioxidants"*. Dr Packer is one of the world's leading researchers on Vitamin E (tocopherols and tocotrienols), alpha lipoic acid, and other biological antioxidants.

Dr. Richard Cutler, PhD., while Head of Gerontology at the Gerontology Research Center (GRC) at the National Institutes of Health, Washington DC, USA, found experimentally that there is a correlation between the concentration of a number of antioxidants in serum with increasing lifespan of mammalian species and that humans had the highest concentration of antioxidants such as vitamin E, Carotenoids and Urate. In simple terms, this means, "<u>The Amount of Antioxidants that You Maintain in Your Body is Directly Proportional to How Long You Will Live</u>."

It's now self-evident from 3 Decades and 30,000 Published Documents, which have shown the link between free radical activity and cell damage, that the balance between your intake of antioxidants and exposure to free radicals may literally be the balance between life and death. You can tip the scales in your favour by simple changes to your diet and antioxidant supplementation.

Our bodies naturally produce some antioxidants, but we are being bombarded increasingly by reactive oxygen species from our environment. Our bodies are literally being overrun. You only have to consider the increasing number of cars over the last few decades and the worldwide public concern over the effect that increasing pollution is having on global warming to know the pollution threat from our environment is increasing. Add to this dilemma the lower quality, and in some cases the toxic nature, of our food, and we don't stand much of a chance!

Fortunately recent scientific studies have begun to identify several antioxidants and their immense value to the human body. There is no miracle antioxidant – you have to have a broad spectrum of antioxidants, many of which work synergistically together in an inter-connected network. There are many kinds of antioxidants available, and hundreds of thousands of clinical studies of the effects of antioxidants on humans have taken place. Also many books and scientific papers have been written on them.

TOP NINE ANTIOXIDANTS

The Top 9 Antioxidants are:

Vitamin E

Vitamin C
Mineral Cofactors – Selenium, Zinc, Copper, and Manganese
Alpha-lipoic Acid
Carotenoids – including Beta-Carotene, Alpha-Carotene, Lutein, Lycopene, Zeaxanthin, Astaxanthin, Beta-Cryptoxanthin
Flavonoids – including Green Tea, Catechins, Bioflavonoids, Grape Seed Extract, Quercetin, Soy Isoflavones
Milk Thistle
Ginkgo Biloba
Coenzyme Q-10

NB. The benefits and characteristics of each of the above antioxidants are described later in this book, under the "1st Pillar of Health – Antioxidants" – see page 80.

Attempting to obtain sufficient levels of antioxidants from our food is becoming increasingly more difficult. Compared to say 50 years ago, food generally has a much lower nutrient content, due to the soil in many cases yielding much less nutrients. This is partly because soil gradually loses its mineral content through over farming, unless the farmer replaces the minerals by adding back mineral-rich manure. But many of the minerals that pass from plant to us are not needed to make the plant grow, so there is no incentive for the farmer to add them back. Between 1939 and 1991 mineral levels in plants have dropped on average by about 22%.

Also many fruits and vegetables are being harvested too early, i.e. before beneficial enzymes have formed and they are being sprayed with chemicals to "preserve and lengthen shelf life as well as to make them look good on the shelves". Much of the "fresh food" we see on the supermarket shelves has been "in storage" for many months and sometimes a year or more! Recent analyses of oranges, which have been stored for a year, have shown a two-thirds drop in nutrient content!

Refining food to make white rice, white flour and white sugar removes up to 90% of the trace minerals. Dr Stephen Davies from London's Bio-Lab Medical Unit analysed 65,000 samples of blood, hair, and sweat over the 15 years up to 1993. Without exception, when the results are compared with the ages of the patients, levels of lead, cadmium, aluminium, and mercury are increasing, while those of magnesium, zinc, chromium, manganese, and selenium are decreasing.

The first group of minerals are toxic – "anti-nutrients" which compete with essential minerals. As we age, those toxic elements accumulate. Today we need more "good" minerals than ever to protect us from the unavoidable toxic minerals, which reach us via polluted food, air, and water!

In the last few years it has been discovered that we can now guarantee, by supplementing with phytonutrients, that we will take in much higher levels of antioxidants than can be obtained from our food. This is achieved by extracting those plant chemicals, which scientific research and randomised double blind placebo controlled clinical studies on humans indicate, can provide much safer protection to the human body than was ever possible in the old days, when man relied solely on the antioxidants which happened to be in his food because he knew no better. Antioxidants are the "Guardians of our Bodies"!

The breakthrough since 1993 in mankind's knowledge of phytochemicals, especially antioxidants, has been described by some as being as significant to the human race as the discovery of antibiotics!

AGEING

Slowing down the ageing process is no longer a mystery. The best results in research studies have consistently been achieved by giving animals low-calorie diets, which are high in antioxidant nutrients – in other words, exactly what they need and no more. This reduces "oxidative stress" and ensures maximum antioxidant protection. "Animals fed in this way not only live up to 40% longer but are also more active during their lives." *(Kotulak, R. and Gorner, P. (editors), "Ageing on hold – Secrets of living Younger Longer," Chapter 5 by R. Walford, 51 – 73: Tribune Publishing, USA, (1992).*

Although long-term studies on humans have yet to be completed, there is every reason to assume that the same principles apply to humans. We all age – it's inevitable! Time stops for no one. But that doesn't mean that we have to let our ageing get the better of us. We <u>can</u> live long, productive lives.

One of the keys to battling ageing is to maintain a positive attitude. You really are as old as you think you are. If you believe that you are young enough to participate in life, then you are. There may be some limitations – you may not have as much energy and your body may not be as flexible – but you can remain active and productive throughout your life.

Another vital aspect of fighting against the negative effects of ageing is to change your viewpoint. We often define ageing in chronological terms. Getting old is measured in the number of years that we have been alive. The truth, though, is that ageing is more a reflection of an accumulation of damage – not an accumulation of years.

Every day that we live we are being bombarded by free radicals. These reactive oxygen species in turn cause damage to our bodies. Ageing, and the problems associated with it, are the result of that accumulated damage from free radicals. As we've already mentioned, antioxidants can go a very long way in helping the body keep away from more than 80 age-related diseases and those diseases can also be treated through antioxidants.

And that's the good news – We don't have to "grow old gracefully" anymore!

We can go kicking and screaming all the way, fighting the very symptoms that claim the lives and productivity of millions of people by simply ensuring that we maintain sufficient levels of antioxidants in our bodies at all times.

THE NEW REVOLUTION

You see, there's a New Revolution taking place out there right now, which is being fuelled by the Ageing Baby Boomers (those born between 1946 and 1964), who are doing everything possible to stay young! People are sick and tired of being sick and tired. We're no longer willing to go to doctors to be told that they're not sure what's wrong, but try this or that drug! We've been placing Band-Aids over problems long enough, now we want the cure!

That cure is primarily antioxidants! Reactive oxygen species or free radicals lead to many of the problems and illnesses we face today. Cancer and Cardiovascular disease are the leading killers in the western world. Yet these two diseases can be treated and in many cases prevented through stopping the damage caused by free radicals in the first place. Other illnesses where free radical damage is implicated, like macular degeneration, diabetes, and the many symptoms associated with ageing, can be prevented, and treated as well, with antioxidants.

Are you ageing prematurely? Will you die prematurely? Will you suffer from degenerative diseases that are so rampant today?

The problem is, and it's a shocking situation, the majority of us are malnourished and immune deficient. But what's even worse – we don't even know or appreciate that fact! Most of us are unaware and simply do not understand that we are in that situation as we keep on "just getting by" day by day! Many people just think, "It won't happen to me!" In adopting that attitude, we are unwittingly taking many unnecessary risks with our health to the potential detriment of our families and ourselves.

Complacency is unwise and unnecessarily dangerous, to say the least. Armed with this new knowledge, we now have so much opportunity to support our health in a simple and easy way through good nutrition! A parallel in the legal world is that "Ignorance is no defence in law"!

On the one hand, people's lack of knowledge, and in some cases complacency, is understandable, because how in our hectic lives, as we "just get by", can we keep pace with all the recent major developments in nutritional science and their benefits to human health?

On the other hand, it makes sense to be open-minded to the new knowledge and also be prepared to be proactive in order to obtain Dynamic Health for the rest of our lives, if that is what we seek!

ARE YOU ONE OF THE MAJORITY – JUST GETTING BY?

IF SO, WILL YOU BE PROACTIVE TOWARDS YOUR HEALTH?

Let's now move on to the Evolution of Scientific Knowledge in this recently developing area of Human Health and Nutrition.

SCIENTIFIC BACKGROUND.

Health Professionals will tell you that the three big behaviour problems are tobacco, diet/obesity, and lack of regular exercise. These are the major risk factors in Cardiovascular disease and Cancer that together are accounting for over 70% of all deaths every year in the Western World.

WHY SUPPLEMENT YOUR DIET?

♦ Lifestyle benefits and lower risk factors come with Dynamic Health, which depends on good nutrition – <u>not</u> when we are "just getting by"!

♦ The Three New Threats to our Health – all Man-Made – are:

   1. Lower mineral content of soil, storage shelf life, and transport are decreasing the nutrient content of our food.

   2. Levels of Toxins are increasing in most areas of our Environment.

   3. Sedentary Lifestyle is putting us out of step with our Evolution.

♦ Antioxidants are the "Guardians of the Body".

"The significant problems we have created cannot be solved at the same level of thinking we were at when we created them". Albert Einstein.

"By giving the body the right molecules, most diseases would be eradicated. Optimum Nutrition is the Medicine of Tomorrow". Dr Linus Pauling – Double Nobel Prize Winner.

"You should make your medicine your food and your food your medicine." Paul Zane Pilzer - <u>The Next Trillion</u>.

<u>In Healthy People, Sub-Optimal Nutrition may result in Vague Symptoms, such as:</u>

Depression, Fatigue, Loss of Appetite, Irritability, Anxiety, Confusion, Mood Swings, Learning difficulties, Insomnia, Poor Concentration, and even Psychosis.
<u>Optimum Nutrition Bible by Patrick Holford – London 1997.</u>

<u>Here are Some Reasons Why those who eat a Nutritious Diet may still need to take Supplements</u>:

Food processing methods and **storage shelf life** strip many nutrients from food.

Smoking **tobacco** and drinking **alcoho**l deplete the body's nutrient stores and displace nutrient intake.

Everyone's biochemistry is unique, what is good for some nutritionally may not be the best for someone else.

Food allergies may affect assimilation of nutrients.

Stress affects body chemistry.

Prescription and over-the-counter medicines may affect absorption of nutrients in the diet and produce side effects.

Poor digestion due to illness, stress, or age-related conditions may not allow your body to make the most of the foods you eat.

Dieting interferes with metabolism; limited intake of foods limits intake of vitamins, minerals and other micro-nutrients.

OVERWHELMING EVIDENCE THAT EVERYONE SHOULD SUPPLEMENT THEIR DIET

"There is not a shred of evidence that diet alone can supply enough micronutrients to attain any level of health above adequate. I've never seen a single study to support the concept that you get everything you need for optimal health from a well-balanced diet." Leibovitz B. – "Nutrition: at the crossroads". Journal of Optimal Nutrition 1992; 1:69 – 83 (USA).

"A National Survey of over 21,500 people showed that *not one of them received 100% of RDA (Recommended Daily Allowance) for 10 basic nutrients from diet alone"*. John Cordaro, President of the Council for Responsible Nutrition, in a testimony before the Sub Committee on Health and Environment of the US House of Representatives on 29th July 1993.

An indication of the serious nutritional deficits being experienced by the general population is provided by a **US Department of Agriculture's Survey** in 1995 of tens of thousands of people. This indicated the percentage of people whose intake from their diet of each critical nutrient, was below Recommended Daily Allowance. (Remember, RDA is the minimum level to avoid deficiency diseases – not for Optimum Nutrition). Some of these are as follows:

- 70% were below the RDA for Calcium and Magnesium,
- 75% were below RDA for the key mineral, Zinc,
- Around 50% were below RDA for the B Vitamins,
- 60% were below RDA for Vitamin A,
- 40% were below RDA for Vitamin C and
- 70% were below RDA for the key antioxidant Vitamin E.

The US Department of Agriculture went on to say, *"only 9% of the population reach the minimum daily intake of essential nutrients. A staggering 91% are deficient"*. But is even reaching the minimum acceptable?

The Need for Supplementation. One of the most significant events in relation to human health and nutrition was the change of mind by one of the most prestigious Medical Institutes in the world, the University of California at Berkeley. Their statement is as follows. *"The Editorial Board of the Wellness Letter has been reluctant to recommend supplementary vitamins* *on a broad scale for healthy people eating healthy diets. But... the accumulation of research in recent years has caused us to change our minds – at least where four vitamins are concerned... These are the 3 so-called antioxidant vitamins, plus the B vitamin folacin... <u>The role these substances play in disease prevention is no longer a matter of dispute</u>.*" – Editorial Board, Univ. of California at Berkeley Wellness Letter, Jan 1994, largest circulation Wellness publication in the World.

The Report "Nutritional Deficiencies in the Netherlands" by Ruud Nieuwenhuis, Director of the Orthomolecular Education Foundation, SOE, was sent to the Dutch Minister of Health, Welfare, and Sport on 10th April 1995. Quote – *"Virtually the entire Dutch population suffers to some extent from nutrition deficiencies of essential vitamins, minerals and trace elements. <u>These deficiencies will inexorably lead to serious health problems</u>.*" **Editor's Note –** *"This study was carried out in the Netherlands only. It is most likely, however, that a similar situation exists in other Western countries."*

"<u>There is overwhelming evidence that a balanced diet is insufficient to meet all nutritional objectives</u>, particularly in the elderly, and that intervention with dietary supplements is necessary for health promotion. This conclusion conflicts with the widely held opinion that people can obtain all of the nutrients they need from eating a balanced diet." Chandra R. K. – "Graying of the Immune system: can nutrient supplements improve immunity in the elderly?" –

Journal of the American Medical Association (JAMA) 1997; 277: 1398 – 1399.

"Almost 90,000 people under the age of 65 die each year. Of these, 32,000 die from Cancer and another 25,000 die each year from heart diseases, strokes, and related diseases. <u>Many of these deaths are related to diet and are preventable</u>." **Department of Health, United Kingdom.**

In a **UK National Food Survey** in 1995 it was found that people in Britain were getting less than the EU RDA (Recommended Daily Allowance) of many of the nutrients measured. This means that the average person in the UK is deficient in most key nutrients when measured against EU RDA, which, remember, is set to avoid deficiency diseases, not for Optimal Health. Some of the deficiencies were as follows:

The average UK Intake of <u>Vitamin C was 13% short of RDA</u>.
The average UK Intake of <u>Iron was 32% short of RDA</u>.
And for <u>Zinc</u>, which is probably the most important mineral we need, the average UK Intake <u>was 49% short of RDA</u>!

"The Myth of the Well-Balanced Diet"

"Part of the problem is propaganda. We are led to believe that as long as you eat a well-balanced diet you get all the nutrients you need. Yet survey after survey shows that even those who believe that they eat a well-balanced diet fail to get anything like the ideal intake of vitamins,

minerals, essential fats, and carbohydrates. It is not easy in today's society, in which food production is inextricably linked to profit. Refining foods makes them last, which makes them more profitable but at the same time deficient in essential nutrients. The food industry has gradually conditioned us to eat sweet foods. Sugar sells, and the more of it we eat the less room there is for less sweet carbohydrates. As our lives speed up we spend less time preparing fresh food and become ever more reliant on ready-meals from companies more concerned for their profit than our health." **The Optimum Nutrition Bible, Part 2, Chapter 7 by Patrick Holford, Founder of the Institute of Optimum Nutrition. Published 1997, London.**

The **American Cancer Society recommends** – *"every adult should consume 5 to 10 servings of fruit and vegetables each day."* However, the average American diet, as well as most other Western diets, contains barely 3 servings of fruits and vegetables daily and one of those is "French Fries"! This is a dangerous daily shortfall. Vegetables and fruit contain the anti-carcinogenic cocktail to which our bodies are adapted. We abandon it at our peril!

The current **Food Pyramids** published by the **US and British Dietetic Associations** recommend that, *"in order to get the Recommended Daily Allowance of vitamins, nutrients, and minerals you need to eat:*

- *2-3 servings of milk, yoghurt, and cheese*
- *2-3 servings of meat, poultry, fish, dry beans, eggs, & nuts*

- *3-5 servings of vegetables*
- *2-4 servings of fruit and*
- *6-11 servings of bread, cereal, rice, and pasta."*

<u>That's a total of 15 to 26 servings a day</u>! To eat all that would mean substantially over-eating, and for many people, it would be nigh impossible. Even then you are likely to obtain only the "low level" RDAs, which were designed to avoid deficiency diseases such as beri beri, rickets, pellagra, and scurvy. So it is clear that the only way to obtain the much higher levels of essential micronutrients for Optimum Health is to supplement your diet.

Dr. Walter C. Willett of Harvard School of Public Health in 2001, put forward new thinking on the recommended daily intakes. His New Food Pyramid modifies the previous ones, above, by separating the good and bad fats and carbohydrates, recommending daily exercise and alcohol in moderation. <u>But his most significant recommendation is "multiple vitamins for most people"</u> because there are many micronutrients and vitamins, such as the powerful antioxidant vitamin E, the optimum doses of which can <u>only</u> be conveniently obtained through supplementation.

"TAKE MULTIVITAMINS", JOURNAL OF THE AMERICAN MEDICAL ASSOCIATION (JAMA), URGES IN POLICY REVERSAL, June 2002.

This is the most significant statement on human nutrition ever made!

They said, quote, ***"Low levels of the antioxidant vitamins (Vitamins A, E & C) may increase risk for several chronic diseases. Most people do not consume an optimal amount of all vitamins by diet alone ... <u>it appears prudent for all adults to take vitamin supplements</u>"*** end quote – JAMA (Journal of the American Medical Association), 19th June 2002. 287:3127-3129.

This is a total reversal of the Journal of the American Medical Association's long-standing anti-vitamin policy since it last made a comprehensive review of vitamins about 20 years ago. **It is now advising all adults to take a multivitamin every day**.

At the time of their <u>previous</u> review of vitamins, JAMA concluded that people of normal health shouldn't take multivitamins because they were a waste of time and money. *"People can get all the nutrients they need from their diet"*, JAMA advised, adding that, *"only pregnant women and chronically sick people may need certain vitamins"*.

The following comments were made on the above Announcement by The Journal of The American Medical Association (JAMA) in June 2002:

> Drs Robert Fletcher and Kathleen Fairfield of Harvard University said, *"Scientists' understanding of the benefits of vitamins has rapidly advanced, and it now appears that people who get enough vitamins may be able to prevent such common chronic*

illnesses as Cancer, heart disease, and osteoporosis".

Jeffrey Blumberg, Chief of Antioxidant Research at Tufts University's Jean Mayer US Dept of Agriculture Human Nutrition Research Center on Aging said, *"It's nice to see this change in philosophy that's saying we can make public-health recommendations based on this really compelling set of data".*

Blumberg said, *"The American Medical Association recommendations underscore a growing concern among nutrition experts that the recommended daily allowances, or RDAs, for many vitamins are set too low. RDAs essentially were established to prevent symptoms of vitamin-deficiency disorders. But evidence is growing that higher levels of many vitamins are necessary to achieve optimum health. <u>The National Academy of Sciences, which sets RDAs, is revising its recommendations based on the new evidence</u>."*

- Fletcher said, *"Even people who eat 5 daily servings of fruits and vegetables may not get enough of certain vitamins for optimum health. Most people, for instance, cannot get the healthiest levels of folate and vitamins D and E from recommended diets. All of us grew up believing that if we ate a reasonable diet that would take care of our vitamin needs. But the new evidence, much of it in the last couple of years, is that vitamins also prevent the usual diseases we deal with every day – heart disease, Cancer, osteoporosis and birth defects."*

- Blumberg said, *"Because foods contain thousands of vitamin-like compounds – many not yet identified – which may be important for good health, vitamin supplements should not be a substitute for a wholesome diet."*

THE 6 "PILLARS OF HEALTH"

Pillars of Health are Nutrient Groupings, which are crucial to our Health.

Our Health is like a building that is dependent on 6 Pillars.

If we are short of one Pillar we are not in very good shape; if we are missing several Pillars, our health is seriously compromised, and if we are missing them all, we're a mess!

The challenge is that our diets will almost certainly be short of nutrients in several Pillars – unless we supplement!

1ˢᵗ PILLAR OF HEALTH – ANTIOXIDANTS.

"Reactive Oxygen Species" or "Free Radicals" are toxic molecules, which alter and damage DNA and cell membranes. They play a major role in ageing. DNA is Deoxyribonucleic acid, which is the main constituent of chromosomes and can reproduce itself. It is the main "life form" and is the key to heredity whereby genetic features can be passed from generation to generation.

In simple terms, **Free Radicals** are unstable toxic molecules, which have an unpaired electron in their orbiting ring. **Antioxidants** are molecules, which can give up an electron from their orbiting ring to a free radical to stabilise it, without themselves turning into a free radical. This stops the damaging chain reaction, which would otherwise lead to premature ageing and many diseases.

We all have millions of abnormal/dead cells in our bodies amongst the trillions of normal cells at any moment in time. Our immune system is designed to neutralise these abnormal cells through its antioxidant defence system. To minimise free radical damage we must have antioxidants and the broadest spectrum the better, continuously circulating in our blood stream in order to maintain effective antioxidant levels in our tissues throughout our bodies every minute of every day of every month of every year.

That broad spectrum of antioxidants is like a mix of instruments in an orchestra, with the very powerful Green Tea Catechins, for example, being the "high decibel" brass section of the orchestra. We need all those antioxidants to develop an interconnected synergistic network of many antioxidants including good levels of Carotenoids, which act as sentinels to that network, for maximum protection.

No single antioxidant protects all body systems; rather, each one provides its own particular benefits, with some providing greater protection to some organs or functions in the body compared to others, while other antioxidants provide more general benefits such as supporting the recycling of other antioxidants.

Several Vitamins and Minerals are Antioxidants and many Phytonutrients (see 2nd Pillar of Health – Phytonutrients – page 113) are also antioxidants such as **Green Tea Catechins**, which are considered the most powerful, followed by the next most powerful which are the Flavonoid **Leucoanthocyanins in Grape Seed extract**.

Antioxidants neutralise Free Radicals and therefore decrease damage caused by Free radicals to cell membranes i.e. the outside of body cells. **Catechins,** however, are a highly specialised class of powerful antioxidant polyphenol flavonoids, <u>which also protect the nucleus and DNA of the cell</u>. **Carotenoids** are also critically important antioxidants because they act as sentinels to the antioxidant network, are the first line of defence and play a crucial role in inter-cell communication. A typical characteristic of Cancer cells is their inability to communicate.

THE TOP 9 ANTIOXIDANTS - Revisited
(Details of each follow)

Vitamin E
Vitamin C
Mineral Cofactors – Selenium, Zinc, Copper, and Manganese
Alpha-lipoic Acid
Carotenoids – Beta-Carotene, Alpha-Carotene, Lutein, Lycopene, Zeaxanthin, Astaxanthin, Beta-Cryptoxanthin
Flavonoids – Bioflavonoids, Green Tea, including Catechins, Anthocyanins, including Grape Seed Extract, Quercetin, and Soy Isoflavones
Milk Thistle
Ginkgo Biloba
Co-enzyme Q10

VITAMIN E

Vitamin E is a collection of 8 different compounds divided into two groups, the tocopherols (d-alpha, beta, gamma & delta) and the tocotrienols. When looking at a Vitamin E supplement, make sure that both these groups are present. These are natural forms of Vitamin E, which are isolated from vegetable oils, which are nearly twice as effective as synthetic Vitamin E, which is made from petrochemicals. Vitamin E is an Essential Vitamin, meaning that our bodies cannot produce it naturally but must ingest it. Vitamin E is one of the most versatile antioxidants and has been linked to most degenerative diseases. It prevents lipid peroxidation in foods and it also helps to prevent the fatty portions of our cells from oxidising. This prevention of oxidation means that the formation of free radicals is stopped, decreasing our risk of disease.

Substantial scientific research, as far back as the 1930s, has proved Vitamin E to be an exceptionally powerful vitamin antioxidant, protecting cells from damage, including Cancer and cardiovascular disease. Indeed it may be the single most important antioxidant when it comes to cardiovascular health. LDL (Low Density Lipoprotein) cholesterol (bad) readily incorporates it resulting in Vitamin E protecting LDLs from free radical damage. Vitamin E also helps reduce LDL cholesterol levels, raises HDL (High Density Lipoprotein) cholesterol (good) levels, inhibits platelet aggregation, and breaks down excess fibrogen. Vitamin E helps the body use oxygen, supports normal blood clotting, protects against thrombosis and atherosclerosis, lowers blood pressure, and helps prevent anaemia. Aside from its antioxidant properties, Vitamin E improves wound healing and helps the repair of damaged tissues and reduces scars. It supports fertility and is associated with healthy nerves, muscle, skin, and hair. Vitamin E can repair and even suppress the damage caused by free radicals. It works synergistically with Vitamin C, as mentioned above. **The Anthocyanins**, part of the Bioflavonoid group, <u>multiply the effect of Vitamin E fifty-fold</u>!

VITAMIN C

Vitamin C (ascorbic acid) strengthens the immune system – fights infections. If you don't get any Vitamin C, you'll come down with scurvy, which causes weakness, anaemia, spongy gums, and bleeding from the mucous membranes.

We lost our capability to produce Vitamin C way back in our evolution. A dog on average produces 3 grams of vitamin C each day, which, bearing in mind that a human being is probably 4 to 5 times the weight of the average dog, puts a major question mark over the RDA (Recommended Daily Allowance) for Vitamin C being only 60mg – only 2% of what a dog produces and only "half of 1%" when adjusted for weight! There are strong grounds for suspicion that this incredibly low EU RDA for Vitamin C is politically or commercially motivated!

In contrast, The Food and Nutrition Board of the US National Academy of Sciences' Institute of Medicine reported, *"available data indicates that very high intakes of vitamin C (2 to 4 grams per day) are well tolerated biologically in healthy mammalian systems"*. While you may not need 2 to 4 grams a day, you should take at least 250mg to see the benefits.

In 1999, Mark Levine reported in the "Journal of the American Medical Association" that, *"Harmful effects have been mistakenly attributed to Vitamin C, including hypoglycaemia, rebound scurvy, infertility, mutagenesis (formation of*

mutations) and destruction of Vitamin B12.
Health Professionals should recognise that
Vitamin C does not produce these effects".

A cold's severity and duration are lessened by as
much as 25% by Vitamin C, which blocks the
action of viral agents but Vitamin C will not
prevent a cold developing. It helps wound
healing and provides support against bruising.
Vitamin C helps form the fibrous connective
tissue, collagen, keeping bones, skin, and joints
firm and strong. It is an antioxidant, detoxifying
pollutants and protecting against Cancer and
heart disease. It has been linked with lowered
cholesterol levels and lowered blood pressure
and promotes more of the good HDL cholesterol,
inhibiting platelet aggregation, and
strengthening blood vessels. Along with Vitamin
E, Vitamin C blocks free radicals in the blood
before they can get to the (bad) LDL cholesterol
molecules. It helps make anti-stress hormones
and turns food into energy and can also act as a
natural anti-histamine agent, reducing the
symptoms of allergies and asthma. Finally
Vitamin C is a great team player, boosting the
work of other antioxidants, especially Vitamin E
and Beta-Carotene. Vitamin C acts to regenerate
these and other nutrients after they neutralise
free radicals. If you maintain good levels of
water-soluble antioxidants, like Vitamin C, and
fat-soluble antioxidants like Vitamin E, then
regeneration will continue effectively. The two
mineral vitamins work together to produce a
synergistic partnership creating greater results
than either can do on their own. Vitamin C also
works with the B vitamins to produce energy.
The Anthocyanins, part of the Bioflavonoid

group, <u>multiply the effect of Vitamin C twenty-fold</u>!

MINERAL CO-FACTORS

Mineral Cofactors. In the natural course of burning oxygen to generate energy, our bodies produce a free radical called **Superoxide.** Superoxide is an oxygen molecule with an unpaired electron and is the most common free radical that our bodies have to deal with. Normally **Superoxide Dismutase**, one of the antioxidant defence systems produced by the body, counteracts Superoxide by catalysing the reaction between two Superoxide molecules and two hydrogen molecules. But if the reaction doesn't happen fast enough, cell walls, mitochondria, and chromosomes – Superoxide's favourite targets – are at risk. This can result in not only death of cells but also in Cancer. Superoxide Dismutase can stop the free radical chain reactions from starting and continuing.

So what does the body need to produce this powerful antioxidant, Superoxide Dismutase? Answer – Mineral Co-factors – specifically Selenium, Zinc, Copper, and Manganese. These minerals are the building blocks that our bodies use to create the antioxidant Superoxide Dismutase enzyme and are described below:

ZINC. Zinc has many different functions all over the body and is a very important mineral antioxidant. It is also an essential building block of one of the body's antioxidant defence system enzymes, Superoxide Dismutase that counteracts Superoxide, the most common free radical the body has to deal with and which comes mostly from the waste oxygen left over by the body's own metabolic processes. (Copper and Manganese (see below) are the other two main building blocks of Superoxide Dismutase.) Zinc is also a component of over 200 enzymes and of DNA and RNA in cell walls and in the production of Vitamin A. Zinc also boosts the immune system, increasing the level of T-lymphocytes, the cells that fight infection. As we age, Zinc levels tend to drop, resulting in many of the problems that we associate with old age. As Zinc levels drop, cells are less and less able to defend themselves and stay healthy. The decline of Zinc in our bodies closely parallels the decline of the immune system. This decline helps to explain why some illnesses seem to strike only the elderly while ignoring the young. Zinc is also essential for growth and healing; it controls sex hormones, supports ability to cope with stress, and promotes a healthy nervous system and brain, especially in the growing foetus. It aids bone and teeth formation, supports wound healing, helps hair to "bloom", and is essential for constant energy.

MANGANESE. Manganese is another essential building block of Superoxide Dismutase. Manganese also promotes healthy bones, cartilage, tissues and nerves, stabilises blood sugar, is important for insulin production, promotes healthy DNA and RNA, is essential for red blood cell synthesis, reduces cell damage and is required for brain function.

COPPER. Copper is also an essential building block of Superoxide Dismutase. Copper supports cardiovascular health. A deficiency of Copper results in oxidative damage to the heart and the liver. When combined with selenium, Copper fights against oxidative damage to the skin and helps prevent anaemia. Copper is relatively easy to obtain from food but it must be in balance with Zinc. An abundance of Copper will deplete Zinc reserves in the body and vice versa. So Copper is essential at the right levels to ensure its "partner", the important mineral Zinc, is able to operate at appropriate levels in the body.

SELENIUM. Selenium is an essential building block of <u>another</u> of the body's antioxidant defence systems, **Glutathione Peroxidase** and has powerful antioxidant properties to help protect against free radicals and carcinogens and it stimulates the immune system. Glutathione Peroxidase works with another enzyme called **Catalase** to remove **"Hydrogen Peroxide"** – another free radical formed naturally in the body. Glutathione Peroxidase also stops the oxidation of fats, especially LDL cholesterol. This means Glutathione Peroxidase helps stop the build-up of plaque in your arteries, meaning better cardiovascular health. Where there is enough Selenium, Glutathione is able to do its job and prevent and repair damage to the cardiovascular system. Selenium also helps Vitamin E strengthen the immune system and thyroid functions and keep the heart, liver, and pancreas healthy. Put Selenium and Zinc together and they help reduce enlarged prostates and improve male sexuality and fertility. Selenium reduces inflammation to fight infections.

ALPHA-LIPOIC ACID

Alpha-Lipoic Acid is an amino acid and a highly significant water and fat-soluble antioxidant found in the body. It is a key antioxidant, which can inhibit the symptoms associated with ageing. Because it is both water and fat soluble, alpha-lipoic acid can go anywhere in the body and help against just about any kind of oxidative damage.

Working synergistically with other antioxidants, especially Vitamins C and E, alpha lipoic acid helps to increase their potency and conserve them. Alpha-lipoic acid also helps increase metabolism while counteracting the oxidation of the metabolic process. This means that the body produces energy more effectively with less damage. It provides cell protection, especially to the main organs of the body, such as the pancreas (insulin production), the liver, the nervous system, and the eyes.

Diabetics should be aware of alpha-lipoic acid's ability to help control blood sugar levels, and to protect against glycation, which causes many of the problems a diabetic can experience. It also helps reduce the level of cholesterol and fight against LDL oxidation. LDL oxidation results in arteriosclerosis, the clogging, and hardening of arteries. The unregulated growth of cells in Cancer can also be halted by alpha-lipoic acid.

By counteracting the effects of oncogene activators – the causes of uncontrolled cell growth – alpha-lipoic acid helps stop the formation of tumours and Cancer. Alpha-lipoic acid also boosts the immune system, the body's defence against Cancer and all types of pathogens. By bonding with toxic metals, including mercury, cadmium, and lead, alpha-lipoic acid also helps detoxify the body. Alpha-Lipoic Acid also provides added protection against allergies, cataracts, chronic fatigue, nervous tissue, and glaucoma. It also provides excellent support to the body when recovering from burns, hepatitis (jaundice), neuropathy (inflammation & deterioration of nerves), and shingles. Alpha-Lipoic Acid is the most synergistic and all-pervasive antioxidant and is key to slowing down the ageing process.

CAROTENOIDS

Carotenoids. Carotenoids are a family of natural fat-soluble nutrients important for antioxidant defence *(Packer, 1992, 1993; Cadenas and Parker, 2002)* found throughout the plant kingdom. Carotenoids give fruits and vegetables their colour. The reds, oranges, yellows, and other bright colours that you see in fruits and vegetables, such as pineapples, citrus fruits, peaches, nectarines, persimmons, tomatoes, papaya, apricots, carrots, watermelons, pumpkins, squashes and sweet potatoes, are caused by the presence of Carotenoids, which are vitally important to our health because they are critical antioxidants. Sometimes their presence is masked by chlorophyll, especially in dark green leafy vegetables like spinach, broccoli, collard greens and kale.

Carotenoids are also ubiquitous across the animal kingdom. They impart colour to many birds (flamingo, ibis, canary, bullfinch, the Egyptian vulture's brightly coloured yellow head), to insects (ladybird), to marine animals (crustaceans, salmon) and flowers.

More than 600 Carotenoids have been identified in nature but less than 50 are abundant in the human diet. Among these, five Carotenoids, Beta-Carotene, Alpha-Carotene, Lycopene, Lutein and Zeaxanthin are found in the blood and known to be important to human health *(Khachik et al., 1992; Gerster, 1993)*. A large number of epidemiological and experimental studies offer strong evidence that Carotenoids are nutritionally important for Normal Cell Regeneration *(Clinton and Giovannucci, 1998; Clinton 1999)*, Eye Health *(Landrum et al., 1997; Cooper et al., 1999)* plus numerous other health aspects linked to unstable oxygen molecules called free radicals *(Rao and Agarwal, 2000; Cadenas and Parker, 2002)*.

In a "Prospective Study of Carotenoids, Tocopherols and Retinol Concentrations and the Risk of Breast Cancer", the authors concluded that Carotenoids may protect against development of Breast Cancer. In women with the highest fifth of Carotenoid concentration, the risk of developing Breast Cancer was approximately half that of women in the lowest fifth for beta-carotene, Lycopene and total carotene. *Cancer Epidemiology Biomarkers &*

Prevention Vol. 11, 451-457, May 2002. Reiko Sato, Kathy J. Helzlsouer, Anthony J. Alberg, Sandra C. Hoffman, Edward P. Norkus and George W. Comstock. Dept. of Epidemiology, Bloomberg School of Public Health, John Hopkins University, Baltimore, Maryland and Dept. of Biomedical Research, Our Lady of Mercy Medical Center, Bronx, New York. USA.

Most of the health benefits of Carotenoids are associated with their action as antioxidants, that is, they protect cells and tissues from the effects of free radicals *(Mortensen et al., 2001; Paiva and Russell, 1999)*. However, certain Carotenoids, such as Alpha and Beta-Carotene are precursors of Vitamin A.

Carotenoids are "sacrificial" antioxidants. In other words, carotenoid molecules are not regenerated like other antioxidants, and are degraded in the process of neutralising reactive oxygen species or free radicals. A typical carotenoid molecule like Lycopene or Beta-Carotene is able to sustain around 20 free radical hits by lipid radicals before it becomes completely destroyed *(Tsuchiya et al., 1994)*. Carotenoids are the first line of defence; they act sacrificially to protect other members of the antioxidant network (such as vitamins E and C) from having to sustain free radical hits. In this way, elevated tissue carotenoid levels will enhance the entire antioxidant network *(Packer, 1994: Packer and Coleman, 1999)* consequently reducing the danger from oxidative stress. Conversely, high levels of oxidative stress (e.g., with smoking) adversely affect the antioxidant network, and the resulting increased free radical activity leads to a depletion or reduction in tissue Carotenoids *(Smidt and Shieh, 2003; Gollnick and Siebenwirth, 2002, Dietrich, 2003; Lee, 1998)*.

Effective antioxidant protection can only be achieved through a powerful interconnected network of dozens of antioxidants. Antioxidants do not exist in isolation – they are intimately linked together insofar that if one breaks, the whole antioxidant network is weakened. <u>Carotenoids, being the first line of defence, act as sentinels of this network and therefore the level of Carotenoids in human tissue is very representative of the strength of the overall antioxidant network</u>.

The critical importance of Carotenoids acting as sentinels of our antioxidant network was scientifically confirmed by Dr. John Bertram, Professor of Cell and Molecular Biology at the John A. Burns School of Medicine and Cancer Research Center at the University of Hawaii, and others. The Report on Dr. Bertram's group's research findings was presented to the BioScience 2004 Conference in Glasgow, Scotland recently – *"University of Hawaii finds link in stopping tumour growth. In a major discovery, chemicals that give vegetables their colour show cancer-fighting properties."*

Dr. Bertram and Marc Goodman, a Researcher at the Cancer Research Center of Hawaii, plus others made the following points in their presentations to the BioScience 2004 Glasgow Conference:

Pigments that give yellow, red and green vegetables their colours stop tumours from growing and can prevent Cancer by keeping cells "talking" to each other.

People who eat large amounts of these vegetables tend to have a lower risk of Cancer and heart and eye diseases.

◆ The study found that these pigments, called Carotenoids, increased the activity of a molecule called Connexin 43.

◆ The Connexin 43 molecule forms small channels between cells and connects nearly all cells in the body. Cells exchange nutrients through the channels and also many signals responsible for normal cellular growth.

◆ But most tumour cells have lost the ability to communicate and become isolated from normal cells.

◆ Treating normal mouse cells with Carotenoids improved communication in the cells and prevented cancer-causing chemicals from forming Cancer.

◆ Communication between cells was also restored when three types of human tumours were treated with Carotenoids. The cells behaved more normally in cultures <u>and</u> when grown in laboratory animals.

◆ *"One of the hallmarks of Cancer is unregulated growth"*, which occurs when

Cancer cells are no longer getting appropriate signals to stop growing.

♦ The research showed that chemicals such as Carotenoids help to regulate growth by ensuring there is communication between cells. As a result, there is "tremendous potential" for types of Carotenoids not only to prevent Cancer, but also to augment Cancer therapy.

♦ Dr. Bertram advises eating Carotenoid-rich vegetables and fruits and is in collaboration with a Biotech Company to develop easily absorbed Carotenoid tablets for use to prevent Cancer, liver and eye disease and damage to the heart.

♦ He said that the researchers looked at five or six Carotenoids and they all appear able to restore communication between cells.

♦ The research also found that the activity of Connexin 43 molecules could be increased by retinoids, another cancer preventative agent derived from vitamin A, especially when combined with Carotenoids.

♦ Dr. Bertram said Carotenoids and Retinoids might stop Cancers from forming by keeping cells communicating. *"Prevention is always better than cure, and prevention of Cancer should be a priority goal for Health Professionals".*

♦ Studies were presented to the BioScience 2004 Conference in Glasgow showing that up to 70% of human Cancer is preventable and 40% could be associated with diet.

♦ Dr. Bertram said that Carotenoid tablets were presently available but they do not dissolve well in water and are not easily absorbed into the body. He is in the process of developing new versions that are much more absorbable.

♦ He said that *"Rapid and more complete absorption of Carotenoids taken by mouth could offer a significant advantage in future Cancer prevention studies"*.

♦ He also said ... *"different Carotenoids accumulate in different tissues. There may be one that is best for Cardiovascular Disease and a different one for Prostate Cancer"*.

This research indicates that we should all consume a broad spectrum of Carotenoids within our overall "orchestra" of antioxidants, regularly, in order to maintain a high concentration of Carotenoids in our body tissues to support our overall antioxidant defence mechanisms.

When the amounts of Carotenoids in the diet are increased, these substances initially accumulate in the lipoproteins in blood *(Smidt et al., 1999)*. Their amount can be increased to double the level. This increase in blood Carotenoids is then reflected in an increase of Carotenoid concentration in all organs in the body, which can take up lipoproteins, including the skin. Thus, the direct measurement of Carotenoids in skin provides information about their levels at "sites of action" all over the body. This is a distinct advantage over measurements of Carotenoids in blood plasma.

Carotenoids help lower the risk of heart disease, certain types of Cancer, enhance the immune system, and protect us from age-related macular degeneration of the eyes. The presence of Carotenoids, as indicated above, also appears to enhance the communication between premalignant cancer cells and normal cells, which can result in normal cells sending growth regulating messages to damaged cells, helping to stop Cancer. Knowledge on other Carotenoids such as Astaxanthin and Beta-Cryptoxanthin is increasing fast.

♦ **ALPHA-CAROTENE.** Alpha-carotene protects against damage to the skin, eyes, liver, and lungs. A close relative of Beta-carotene, Alpha-carotene has many of the same characteristics, whilst also being very effective in the fight against Cancer.

♦ **BETA-CAROTENE**. For decades, Beta-Carotene was considered significant only as a precursor to Vitamin A. This began to change when the U.S. National Academy of Sciences' Diet, Nutrition, and Cancer Studies suggested that diets high in Beta-Carotene reduced the risk of heart disease and many forms of Cancer. Vitamin A, which is Retinol and comes from Beta-carotene as and when the body needs it, is oil soluble and can be stored in the liver. By providing the body with much of the Vitamin A it needs through Beta-Carotene, the unlikely overdosing of Vitamin A is no longer an issue. Beta-

Carotene is needed for healthy skin, inside and out, protecting against infections. An important antioxidant, it boosts the immune system, and is essential for night vision.

♦ **LUTEIN**. The Journal of the American Medical Association (JAMA) published in November 1994 a study on the role of Carotenoids in preventing macular degeneration of the eyes, which affects 37% of those over 75. Lutein and another carotenoid named Zeaxanthin were found to give the most protection against macular degeneration. Lutein helps protect the fat within the eye cells from oxidation. The body can make Zeaxanthin from Lutein, so it is important to take in sufficient Lutein. Lutein also helps in the fight against Cancer by increasing the amount of time tumours take to appear, increasing white cell growth, and decreasing tumour cell growth.

♦ **LYCOPENE**. Tomato products have been linked to the prevention of certain types of Cancer. Research at Harvard University showed that men who ate tomato-based products had up to a 45% less chance of developing prostate cancer. What is it in tomatoes that protects against Cancer? – Lycopene. Lycopene gives tomatoes their red colour. Scientific studies also show that people who eat tomato products are less likely to get Cancer of the mouth, oesophagus, and digestive tract. Research also indicates that Lycopene is twice as effective as Beta-Carotene in reducing oxidative damage and Lycopene has also been shown to increase the resistance of bad LDL cholesterol to oxidation – a major factor in arteriosclerosis.

FLAVONOIDS

Another very significant group of phytochemical antioxidants is the **Flavonoid** Group. They are powerful Antioxidants, are rapidly absorbed, and some stay up in the blood for as long as 3 days. The Flavonoids that are important antioxidants are the **Bioflavonoids, Green Tea, including Catechins, Grape Seed Extract, Quercetin, and Soy Isoflavones.**

BIOFLAVONOIDS are found in the rind of many citrus fruits and in vegetables. Rather than a single chemical, bioflavonoids are a collection of substances with similar structures. Bioflavonoids can be divided into 12 groups – the most important are marked * below:

- Anthocyanins *
- Anthocyanidins
- Leucoanthocyanins incl. Grape Seed Extract *
- Flavones
- Flavonols
- Flavonones
- Flavonolols
- Isoflavones (good source – Soy) *
- Chalcones
- Dihydrochalcones
- Aurones
- Catechins (mainly from Green Tea) *

Bioflavonoids are characterised by their antioxidant actions and the food that produces them. To coin a phrase, "it's all bioflavonoids". Aside from their abilities as antioxidants, bioflavonoids provide other health benefits. They help detoxify the body, reducing levels of metals that can cause more free radicals. Bioflavonoids also help stabilise collagen, giving you healthier skin, tendons, cartilage, and muscle. Enzymes that are involved in viral replication, cataracts, asthma, and allergies are all inhibited by bioflavonoids. It is important to take in a wide range of bioflavonoids to maximise benefits. Some bioflavonoids can also cross the blood-brain barrier to reach brain tissue, which is highly susceptible to oxidative damage. Not even the most powerful antibiotic can reach the brain! Citrus Bioflavonoids help vitamins C and E to work, strengthen capillaries, and speed up healing of wounds, sprains, and muscle injuries.

◆ **GREEN TEA**. Green Tea is a very popular Asian drink. Green Tea is the antiviral – anticancer antioxidant. Green Tea lowers cholesterol and blood pressure, blocks carcinogens, inhibits bacteria and viruses, neutralises harmful fats and oils and protects against ulcers. Green Tea contains a combination of bioflavonoids that are beneficial to your health and act as preventatives to different diseases. The combination of several bioflavonoids, vitamins, and minerals – all working synergistically – makes green tea a very powerful antioxidant nutrient.

In addition to its powerful antioxidant properties, recent research suggests that Green Tea Extract, including high levels of Catechins, may also provide other highly significant health benefits, by helping to reduce heart disease risk factors known as Metabolic Syndrome X or Insulin Resistance Syndrome. These terms are used to describe a group of heart disease risk factors, including high levels of abdominal fat and bad cholesterol, high blood pressure, and abnormal glucose metabolism. These symptoms are thought to run in families with a history of Type 2 diabetes. Researchers anticipate that clinical trials on humans will show that Green Tea, including its Catechins, is highly beneficial in protecting against and helping to reduce the effects of Metabolic Syndrome X and Insulin Resistance Syndrome.

♦   **CATECHINS** – especially Epigallocatechin gallate (EGCg). Out of the 5 Catechins, Epigallocatechin (EGC) and Epigallocatechin gallate (EGCg) are two of the most powerful free radical scavengers known to man. EGCg, in particular, has the ability to protect the nucleus and DNA of body cells rather than just the cell membrane. It has been scientifically proven by sixty or more in-vitro research studies by independent institutions in several countries to induce apoptosis of many types of human cancer cells, i.e. kill them. (For details of 7 of those Research Studies, see 2nd Pillar – Phytonutrients – page 113).

♦   **ANTHOCYANINS**. The Anthocyanins, listed above, can increase the potency of vitamin E by around 50-fold and Vitamin C by around 20-fold. *"They are the most powerful, natural Free-Radical Scavengers yet discovered."* Metagenics, 1994.

♦   **GRAPE SEED EXTRACT**. Grape Seed Extract with Leucoanthocyanin also includes proanthocyanidins. Grape Seed Extract promotes healthy skin, blood vessels, and soft-tissue healing. It also scavenges free radicals in the brain because it is one of several bioflavonoids that can cross the blood-brain barrier to reach brain tissue, which is highly susceptible to oxidative damage. Additionally, Grape Seed Extract enhances the effectiveness of other antioxidants, especially Vitamins C and E, and protects the body against the effects of radiation, pesticides, pollution, and heavy metals.

♦ **QUERCETIN.** Quercetin is a powerful bioflavonoid found in onions, cayenne pepper, garlic, and green tea. Working as an antioxidant, Quercetin stops the production of free radicals. It also prevents free radicals from oxidising bad LDL cholesterol. Oxidised LDL cholesterol is a precursor to arterial damage and arteriosclerosis. Quercetin also helps detoxify the body of excessive amounts of iron and works against "abnormal, sticky" platelets – two factors thought to be significant factors in arteriosclerosis.

♦ **SOY ISOFLAVONES**. Soy contains a balance of the essential amino acids that your body needs, making it a great source of protein. Soy also contains an isoflavone called **"Genestein"**. Genestein inhibits the growth of cancer cells. Several scientific studies have shown that Genestein blocks prostate and breast cancer growth. Soy has also been shown to lower cholesterol and help to prevent heart disease. It will also help prevent cataracts, maintain healthy kidneys, reduce diabetic need for insulin, and help to prevent osteoporosis.

MILK THISTLE

Milk Thistle. To most people Milk Thistle is a weed that can quickly take over the garden! But did you know that Milk Thistle can detoxify the liver in cases of cirrhosis, hepatitis, jaundice, and the effects of alcohol and drug abuse. The active ingredient in Milk Thistle is Silymarin that is a group of flavonoid compounds, which have a remarkable ability to protect the liver from oxidative damage while enhancing the liver's ability to detoxify the body. Silymarin seems to be very specific in its antioxidant activity in the liver.

One of the ways in which Silymarin helps the liver is by preventing the depletion of glutathione – an important enzyme linked to the liver's ability to detoxify. Reduction of Glutathione reserves leaves liver cells vulnerable to damage. A healthy liver is vital to fighting the many contaminants that enter our body through the environment. Many carcinogens, like air and water pollutants, nicotine and alcohol, are broken down by the liver. A healthy liver is vital in today's contaminant-rich world. As an antioxidant, Silymarin protects liver cells from free radicals. In addition to treating liver problems, Milk Thistle can also support the digestive system.

GINKGO BILOBA

Ginkgo Biloba is the oldest living tree species on the earth. It is also one of the few plants that are "sexual" – the male flowers are found on one plant while the female fruits are on a different one. "Biloba" means that the leaves have two lobes, like two Japanese fans held together. Ginkgo is particularly helpful in increasing blood flow in the smallest blood vessels – capillaries. By opening up the capillaries to blood flow; toxins are washed out of the body. However, if these toxins are allowed to build up, free radical levels also rise. This will result in damage to the capillaries as well as to the organs that they feed.

Ginkgo has been used in Asia for over a thousand years. It has been used to treat asthma, help digestion, prevent drunkenness, ease bladder irritation and revive sexual energy and is also used as an energy booster.

Many studies have been done detailing ginkgo's effect on the brain. The brain ages just as the rest of the body does, but it may be able to regenerate itself to some extent. The best way to maintain brain health is to constantly challenge the organ – stay mentally active and avoid becoming a couch potato. In October 1997, a study published in "The Journal of the American Medical Association" reported that Ginkgo improved cognitive performance in some patients.

Ginkgo also helps to ease symptoms of asthma and allergies. When reacting to allergens, your body will secrete a chemical called PAF. Often, the body will overreact, increasing the symptoms of the allergy. The same holds true for asthma, but ginkgo blocks the activation of this chemical, PAF, relieving these symptoms.

Eye damage can also benefit from ginkgo. A Swedish study showed that ginkgo improved the vision of people suffering from retinal degeneration. A leading cause of macular degeneration is the haemorrhaging of the tiny blood vessels of the eye, usually due to oxidative damage. By strengthening these tiny blood vessels and by acting as an antioxidant, ginkgo helps counteract eye disease. A great advantage of taking Ginkgo for the eyes along with other supplements, including Lutein and Zeaxanthin, is because Ginkgo enables the other active ingredients to pass through the tiny blood vessels in and around the eyes, allowing their benefits to be delivered right into the cells of the eyes.

Ginkgo also has the ability to enable other nutrients to be delivered right into the cells of all the other extremities of the body, including the ears.

CO ENZYME Q 10

Co-enzyme Q10 (Co Q10), which is produced by the body, exerts a central control in your energy system, improves heart function and other cardiovascular functions, helps to normalise blood pressure, increases exercise tolerance, is an antioxidant, and boosts immunity – an incredibly important nutrient! Co Q10 is almost a vitamin. It works and acts just like a vitamin but it has never been awarded that title.

Co Q10 is ubiquitous throughout your body – it's literally in every cell – hence its other name, **Ubiquinone.** Our bodies cannot function without it. Energy couldn't be produced without Co Q10, which is responsible for energy in two ways. Firstly, Co Q10 helps create at least three of the enzymes used for ATP (Adenosine TriPhosphate), the fuel that is released through hydrolysis in the cell mitochondria and burned for energy, to create ADP (Adenosine DiPhosphate). Secondly, Co Q10 creates energy directly by playing a role in electron and proton transfer as energy passes through the mitochondrial wall and the cell wall.

Unfortunately, believe it or not, your body starts cutting back on the production of Co Q10 when you are about 20 years old! This makes additional intake of Co Q10 very important. Co Q10 can be found in various foods, or it can be taken as a supplement. If you want to obtain it from your diet, about a pound of sardines, two pounds of liver, or 2.5 pounds of peanuts will yield around 30 milligrams, which is only 20 to 30% of your body's recommended requirement of 100 to 150 milligrams a day – so supplementing makes far more sense! Of course, your body can make its own Co Q10, but the process has 17 stages involving 8 vitamins and several trace elements, which leaves a lot of room for something to go wrong! Low levels of selenium also result in a drop in Co Q10, while increased levels of the B vitamins raise it.

Co Q10 does more than provide energy for your body. Mechanically speaking, heart failure occurs when the muscle responsible for pulling blood into the heart stops doing its job. The heart then runs out of oxygen, loses its tight muscle tone, and begins to relax. This causes the heart to enlarge, making it more difficult to pull blood in. As it becomes more difficult to pull in blood, blood pressure increases and the heart begins working even harder. If this continues, there may be an electrical blowout called a myocardial infarction or heart attack. Co Q10 makes the heart pump more blood with each beat, causing the heart rate to drop and the muscle size to decrease. Co Q10 also lowers the level of LDL cholesterol, reducing the risk of arteriosclerosis and oxidative damage.

The immune system also benefits from Co Q10, which, when given to elderly people, stimulates the production of antibodies by 2.5 times and restores the immune system to about 80% of its original potency.

A Polish study has shown that Co Q10 supplements can help to prevent oxidative damage to the brain. Lesions and neurological damage caused by spasms of the blood vessels in the brain are usually the result of free radical damage. This can lead to memory loss, stroke, and Cancer. Co Q10 can reduce the risk of all these by controlling oxidative damage.

So a summary of the crucial benefits of maintaining healthy levels of Co Q10 in the body, bearing in mind the body's production of Co Q10 starts falling from the age of 20, are as follows:

1. Energy generation in <u>every cell</u> in the body.
2. Support of the <u>cardiovascular system</u> by protecting against congestive heart failure, angina pectoris, cardiac arrhythmias, high blood pressure, and arteriosclerosis.

3. Prevention and support in cases of breast, lung, colon, prostate, and other types of <u>Cancer</u>.
4. Support in cases of <u>muscular dystrophy and periodontal disease</u>.
5. Protection against <u>free radical damage</u> to all our body cells.
6. <u>Slowing of the ageing process</u>.

OTHER ANTIOXIDANTS

N-acetyl-L-Cysteine (NAC), a sulphur containing amino acid, supports kidney function and is needed for glutathione production. **Glutathione** also helps maintain Glutathione Peroxidase, an important antioxidant enzyme that is part of the body's antioxidant defence system, at adequate levels in the cells.

Other Flavonoid Antioxidants include, Bilberry, Cat's Claw, Cranberry, Hawthorn, Liquorice, Oligomeric Proanthocyanidins, including Pycnogenol, St John's Wort, and Uva-Ursi (Bearberry). Each provides specific health benefits to the body in addition to being antioxidants.

There are also many other antioxidants such as Burdock, Capsicum (cayenne/peppers), Cordyceps Sinensis, Curcumin (Turmeric), Garlic, Ginger, Melatonin (hormone), Methionine (amino acid), Nicotinamide Adenine Dinucleotide with high-energy hydrogen (NADH – also known as Coenzyme 1, a form of Vitamin B3)), Siberian Ginseng, Schisandra. Again, each of these provides specific health benefits to the body in addition to being antioxidants.

RESEARCH STUDIES ON ANTIOXIDANTS

A Major Conference on Antioxidant Vitamins and Beta-Carotene in Disease Prevention took place in London in October 1989. 11 countries, namely USA, UK, Canada, Germany, France, Japan, Italy, Austria, Switzerland, Finland and South Africa were represented. Many highly respected and famous Medical Institutions, such as the US National Cancer Institute, US National Institute on Ageing, John Hopkins, Tufts University, Columbia University, and many others took part.

The report on that Conference took 15 months to produce and included 207 pages and 1373 references. It was published as a Supplement to Volume 53, No.1 (January 1991) of the American Journal of Clinical Nutrition. This started to change people's thinking on the protective power which antioxidant vitamins and beta-carotene could provide to the human body.

Vitamin E lowers risk of Heart Attack. At an American Heart Association's Annual Meeting, the Harvard School of Public Health reported two major studies indicating that taking Vitamin E Supplements reduces the risk of heart disease:

1. 87,245 Female Nurses: Those taking Vitamin E supplements for more than 2 years had a 46% lower risk of heart attack.

2. 51,529 Male health Professionals: Those taking Vitamin E supplements for more than

2 years had a 37% lower risk of heart disease.

3. <u>The amount of Vitamin E in vitamin-rich foods was not enough to produce protection</u>.

4. Reduced heart attack risk only occurred when people took Vitamin E supplements of at least 100 I.U. each day.

At the First Joint Conference on Healthy Ageing, held by the World Health Organisation and the United Nations in April 1996, *"They concurred that antioxidants, including <u>vitamins E and C, Carotenoids and Alpha-lipoic acid</u>, when taken in supplementary form can help to protect the body from free radicals."*

"There certainly is reason to think that <u>Glutathione</u> may play a role in macula degeneration (of the eye)". **Paul Sternberg, M.D., Ophthalmology Times, 15th June 1996**.

Research by Clark et. al. into the benefits of Selenium, which was published in the Journal of the American Medical Association (JAMA) on 25th December 1996, showed that

"in those who were taking 200 mcg per day of Selenium, which is 5 times the US daily consumption, there was a reduction in the overall incidence of Cancer of 42%, and a reduction in Cancer mortality of 50%".

As part of the Proceedings of the National Academy of Sciences on the 19th March 1996, Malins et. al., at the Pacific Northwest

Research Foundation, Seattle, WA reported that

"DNA from Invasive Cancers contains twice as much Free Radical Damage as DNA from Contained Cancers." Also *"Free Radicals induce DNA Disorder which changes Contained Cancer to Invasive Cancer."* Malins' suggestions were *"Test patients for Radical-Induced DNA disorders and <u>treatment should include antioxidants.</u>"*

A Commentary on Malins by Russel J. Reiter, University of Texas Health Science Center, San Antonio, Texas said *"There is a need for Antioxidants which can enter Cancer cells in sufficient amounts to provide "On-Site" defense of DNA, and there may be a requirement for several antioxidants in combination."*

On 15th March 1996 the results of Cancer Research by Susan J Duthie et al. at the Rowatt Research Institute, Aberdeen, Scotland were published. Half the 100 subjects were controls and the other half, of which 50% were smokers, had white blood cells exposed to the Hydroxyl Radical. **Result**: There was one third less Free Radical damage in the Antioxidant Group, which had been taking a combination of Beta Carotene, Vitamin C, and Vitamin E. <u>This is the first study that has shown</u> *<u>"A highly significant moderating effect of long-term Antioxidant Supplementation on oxidative DNA damage"</u>*.

"Recognising the important role of some vitamins and minerals <u>beyond that of preventing deficiency...</u> **the National Academy of Sciences**

in the USA, in contrast with past practices, *is now considering use of evidence for decreasing risk of chronic disease in settling RDAs... Evidence is rapidly accumulating, that intakes above the RDA for some micronutrients, provide benefits in reducing the risk of chronic disease..."* – **John N. Hathcock, American Journal of Clinical Nutrition, 1994.**

There is now convincing scientific evidence that to obtain Dynamic Health it is necessary to take in 5 to 10 times the RDAs (which are essentially minimums) of many micronutrients!

2nd PILLAR OF HEALTH – PHYTONUTRIENTS.

Phytonutrients are chemical compounds found in plants that possess certain nutritional qualities unique to the plants they are derived from. They are whole foods in fruits and vegetables that can prevent disease. *"Just a few years ago, scientists didn't know phytochemicals existed. But today they are the new frontier in cancer-prevention research."* – **Newsweek, USA, 25th April 1994.**

Examples of Phytonutrients are Astragalus, Bilberry, Black Cohosh, Broccoli/Cabbage/Cauliflower (Sulforafane), Capsicum (Cayenne), Cat's Claw, Chamomile, Cordyceps, Cranberry, Dong Quai, Echinacea, Evening Primrose, Feverfew, Garlic, Ginger, Ginkgo biloba, Ginseng Panax, Ginseng Siberian, Goldenseal, Grape Seed, Green Tea, Hawthorn, Horse Chestnut, Indole 3-carbinol, Kava Kava, Liquorice, Marigold (Lutein), Milk Thistle, Red Yeast Rice, Reishi, Saw Palmetto, Schisandra, Soy Isoflavones (Genistein), St John's Wort, Tomato (Lycopene), Turmeric Root (Curcumin), Uva-Ursi, Valerian, Vitex (Chasteberry).

Each of these Phytonutrients supports specific Human Biological Systems and Activities and several of them also provide Antioxidant Protection to the Human Body.

RESEARCH STUDIES ON PHYTONUTRIENTS

CATECHINS. Recent significant research within the whole area of Phytonutrients relates to **Catechins,** which are Green Tea Polyphenols, part of the large family of Bioflavonoids. <u>**Catechins are amongst the most potent antioxidants and protect DNA and the nucleus of the cell**</u>. These are:

- Epigallocatechin (EGC)
- Epicatechin (EC)
- **Epigallocatechin gallate (EGCg)**
- Gallocatechin gallate (GCg)
- Epicatechin gallate (ECg)

Of these catechins, the **Epigallocatechins (especially EGCg)** appear to have the greatest capacity to quench free radicals. <u>EGCg is 100 times more powerful than Vitamin C and 25 times more powerful than Vitamin E at protecting cellular DNA according to Kansas University, USA</u>.

Out of a Total of over 60 Studies, there now follow 7 Verbatim Extracts from Independent Research Studies in several countries into the Antioxidant Power of the Green Tea Catechin "Epigallocatechin gallate" (EGCg):

1. <u>**Chemo Protection**</u>**: A Review of the Potential Therapeutic Antioxidant Properties of Green Tea (Camellia sinensis) and certain of its Constituents.**

Introduction: *"With serious and comparatively intractable diseases such as Cancer, the wisest policy would seem to be to provide a greater emphasis on prevention rather than to attempt to find cures after the disease has become established."*

Conclusions: *"There is a large and growing body of recent evidence that green tea, probably because of its content of polyphenolics, most particularly Epigallocatechin gallate (EGCg) possesses anti-tumour properties. The huge worldwide consumption and apparent lack of toxicity, except in specific populations (end stage renal disease, for example), lead to the cautious recommendation that the material does little harm and may well do significant good and can be supported as an adjunctive therapy to the employment of a good diet, exercise and avoidance of high risk behaviour. Further clinical studies are badly needed."*

Lester A. Mitscher, Michel Jung, Delbert Shankel, Jin-Hui Dou, Linda Steele and Segaran P. Pillai at Departments of Medicinal Chemistry and Microbiology and Genetics, Kansas University, Lawrence, Kansas. USA. Grant Sponsors National Institutes of Health and the National Cancer Institute. Medicinal Research Reviews, Vol. 17, No. 4, 327 – 365 (1997).

2.   *"The important features of Epigallocatechin gallate (EGCg) and green*

tea as cancer preventatives in humans are as follows: they are non-toxic, they have a wide range of target organs and they have inhibitory effects on the growth of cancer cells."

A.Komori et al — Anticarcinogenic activity of Green Tea Polyphenols on human lung cancer cell line, PC-9, Japan J. Cancer Res. 88 (1997) 639 — 643. Saitama Cancer Centre Research Institute, Japan. 22nd July 1997.

3.   *"Green Tea Epigallocatechin gallate (EGCg) shows a pronounced growth inhibitory effect on human colorectal and breast cancerous cells. It also induced a significant amount of apoptosis (programmed cell death) in the cancerous cells (i.e. killed them) but did not have that effect on their normal counterparts."*

Zong Ping Chen et al, Dept. of Chemistry, and Chi-Tang Ho et al, Centre for Advanced Food Technology Rutgers, the State University of New Jersey. 24th March 1998.

4.   *"Green Tea constituent EGCg is shown to induce apoptosis (death) of Human Epidermoid Carcinoma cells, Human carcinoma keratinocytes and Human Prostate Carcinoma cells. The research also suggested that Green Tea may reduce the risk in humans associated with cancers of the bladder, prostate, oesophagus and stomach."*

N. Ahmad et al, Dept. of Dermatology, A-L. Nieminen, Dept. of Anatomy, School of Medicine, Case Western Reserve University, Cleveland, Ohio. 9th October 1997. This work was supported by grants from the National Cancer Institute, National Institutes of Health, Dept. of Health & Human Services and the Breast Cancer Fund of California.

5. *"Induction of apoptosis (programmed cell death) in Human Prostate Cancer cell lines LNCaP, PC-3 and DU 145 by the Green Tea component, Epigallocatechin gallate (EGCg)."*

A. Paschka, R Butler, Dept. of Urology and C. Young, Dept. of Biochemistry and Molecular Biology, Mayo Clinic/Foundation, Rochester, MN, 25th February 1998. This work was supported by grants from the U.S. National Institute of Health and the National Cancer Institute.

6. *"Why drinking Green Tea could prevent Cancer. Human Cancers need proteolytic enzymes to invade cells and form metastases. One of these enzymes is urokinase (uPA). Inhibition of uPA can decrease tumour size and even cause complete remission of Cancers in mice. Research showed that Green Tea Polyphenols, especially EGCg, showed good inhibitory potential. EGCg's ability to inhibit uPA compared with that of the well known inhibitor, Amiloride, showed that*

EGCg was weaker but can be consumed in much higher doses without toxicological effects. The maximum dose of Amiloride is 20mg a day, whereas a single cup of green tea contains 150mg of EGCg and some people drink 10 cups a day! Such high levels of a uPA inhibitor are likely to have a physiological effect and could reduce incidence of Cancer in humans or the size of cancers already formed. Theoretically, EGCg might inhibit cancer formation in many ways; however we postulate that the well-known anti-cancer activity of green tea is driven by inhibition of uPA, one of the most frequently over-expressed enzymes in human cancers."

J. Jankun & S. Selman, Dept. of Urology and R Swiercz, Dept. of Physiology and Molecular Medicine, Medical College of Ohio, Toledo, OH. Nature, Vol. 387, 5th June 1997, Page 561.

7.   ***"How Green Tea prevents Cancer".*** **This paper was presented to the 38th Annual Meeting of the American Society for Cell Biology, 12th to 16th December 1998 in San Francisco.**

"The research team studied an enzyme located on the surface of many cancer cells including Breast, Prostate, Colon and Neuroblastome. This enzyme, named quinol (NADH) oxidase, or NOX, not only functions as an oxidase but also carries out thioldisulfide interchanges among cell surface proteins. NOX activity is required *for growth, in both normal and cancerous cells. Normal cells are careful to express the NOX enzyme only when they are dividing – for example, in response to growth hormone signals. In contrast, cancer cells have somehow gained the ability to express NOX activity at all times. This overactive form of NOX, known as tNOX (tumour-associated NOX), is very important for the growth of cancer cells, since drugs that inhibit tNOX activity also block tumour cell growth in culture."*

The team's important new finding was that – *"EGCg inhibits the tNOX activity of cancer cells – in other words, at low doses. Importantly, EGCg does not inhibit the NOX activity of healthy cells. In parallel studies of living cells, they found that EGCg inhibits the growth of, and kills cancerous human mammary (BT-20) cells in culture, but does not kill cultured, non-cancerous human mammary (MFC-10A) cells."*

"The analysis of blood serum from patients suggests that tNOX activity is broadly, if not universally, associated with human Cancer. The tNOX protein is anchored in the outer leaflet of the surface membrane, and is shed into the bloodstream, since tNOX is present in serum samples from cancer patients. In contrast, drug-responsive tNOX is not found in the sera of healthy volunteers."

"This work is important for several reasons:

I. *It shows that green tea infusions and EGCg, an active "principle" in green tea, both inhibit an enzyme required for cancer cell growth, and can kill cancer cells with no ill effect on healthy cells.*

II. *tNOX assays can now be used to test the relative potency of different kinds of tea and tea chemicals, against cancer cells in culture.*

III. *It provides a rational scientific basis for the use of tea infusions (tea drinking) to slow the growth of cancer cells.*

IV. *Last, but certainly not least, drinkers of green tea worldwide will be heartened to know that the health benefits of their daily routine has finally attracted the attention of cancer biologists!"*

Andrew Bridge, Pelchuan Sun, Lian-Ying Wu, Dorothy M Morre, and D. James Morre, Departments of Medicinal Chemistry & Molecular Pharmacology, and Foods & Nutrition, Purdue University, West Lafayette, Indiana 47907 USA, December 1998.

In addition to **Green Tea's** powerful antioxidant properties, recent research on animals is suggesting that it may help reduce risk factors for heart disease, including bad cholesterol and high blood pressure. Tegreen 97, a derivative of Green Tea, improved glucose and lipid metabolism in obese rats that had features similar to Metabolic Syndrome X. Tegreen 97 also enhanced insulin sensitivity, and balanced the metabolic rate of fat deposit and fat burning. Researchers anticipate that clinical trials on humans will show that Tegreen 97 is highly beneficial in assisting the body processes that can get out of control resulting in Metabolic Syndrome X, a term used to describe a group of heart disease risk factors, including high levels of abdominal fat and bad cholesterol, high blood pressure, and abnormal glucose metabolism. Also known as Insulin Resistance Syndrome, the symptoms are thought to run in families with a history of Type 2 diabetes.

H Yu, Z Zhu, W Yin, J-S Zhu of Pharmanex Beijing Pharmacology Center and Provo, Utah. Presented to Annual Meeting of American Physiological Society held at San Diego Convention Center, 11-15 April 2003.

REISHI. There has also been some recent research into another very significant Phytonutrient, <u>Reishi *(Ganoderma lucidum)*, indicating that it inhibits the invasiveness of Breast and Prostate Cancer Cells</u>. Breast Cancer is the most common malignancy in women in the United States, accounting for 33% of all Cancers diagnosed in females. Also, Prostate Cancer is one of the principle Cancers of men in the West!

Recent in vitro and animal studies have suggested that Reishi *(Ganoderma lucidum)*, in the form of a dietary supplement, ReishiMax GLp® exhibits anticancer activity, mainly through the stimulation of the host immune system by polysaccharides or by the cyto-toxic effects of triterpenes. They demonstrated that purified spores or fruiting body of Reishi *(Ganoderma lucidum)* down-regulated the expression of the enzyme urokinase plasminogen activator (uPA) and uPA receptor (uPAR), which resulted in the suppression of cell motility in both Breast and Prostate Cancer cells. One of the studies investigated how Reishi *(Ganoderma lucidum)* can modulate the metastatic behaviour of the highly invasive human breast Cancer cells MDA-MB-231.

The data in the study demonstrated that *Ganoderma lucidum* inhibits cell adhesion, cell migration, and cell invasion of highly metastatic breast Cancer cells. Furthermore, *Ganoderma lucidum* suppressed the anchorage-independent growth (colony formation) of MDA-MB-231 cells.

Based on these results, Reishi – *Ganoderma lucidum* – may contribute to reducing invasion and metastasis (spreading) of breast and prostate Cancers by inhibiting Cancer cell adhesion, cell migration, cell invasion, and growth of Cancer cells.

Using *Ganoderma lucidum* in the form of a dietary supplement such as ReishiMax GLp®, without extraction or purification steps, could possibly increase the biological effects of *Ganoderma lucidum*. Furthermore, this application is in accord with the practice of herbal medicine, in which the use of the whole product could reduce the toxicity of its purified components, and the interaction between different biologically active components can increase the therapeutic activity of the whole product.

The scientists say that since *Ganoderma lucidum* is currently available in the form of a dietary supplement – ReishiMax GLp® – the clarification of its potential anti-cancer activity would scientifically justify its use by Cancer patients. They also say that the supplement, ReishiMax GLp® could have preventive effects against secondary metastases, which are responsible for the high mortality of invasive Breast and Prostate Cancer.

Veronika Slivova, BS; Tatiana Valachovicova, BS; Jiahua Jiang, PhD; Daniel Sliva, PhD at The Cancer Research Laboratory, Methodist Research Institute, Department of Medicine, School of Medicine, Indiana University (DS), Indianapolis, Indiana, United States. Winter 2004.

Phytonutrients Generally.

As mentioned earlier there are over 300 Phytonutrients, which are known to be beneficial to the human body. They are too numerous to mention each of them here. Suffice it to say a good number are needed on a daily basis to provide a broad spectrum of general antioxidants for the whole population. However, many phytonutrients are scientifically proven to provide benefits to specific parts of the body in the general population, in addition to their antioxidant benefits, such as Lycopene, the most potent Carotenoid antioxidant that has far-reaching cell-protective (prostate) and anti-ageing benefits, Lutein, another Carotenoid, for protecting the retina and macular area of the eye and Co Enzyme Q10 for protection of the Cardiovascular system and the heart in particular, and energy production. Another, such as Saw Palmetto, is male specific for promoting Prostate health. (See "Carotenoids" – page 90 for details of some Research Studies on Carotenoids, especially relating to their important support of Cell Communication.)

The Institute of Natural Product Research (INPR) of Marine on St. Croix, MN, USA produced "Natural Dietary Supplements: A Desktop Reference" in September 1998. It includes Monographs on Botanical and Dietary Supplements. This is a unique publication, which provides Health Professionals with all the information they need on each natural botanical phytonutrient to the same degree of detail as they have on prescription drugs.

Each "Botanical Phytonutrient Monograph" includes – a **"Safety Profile Section"**, which sets out **"Side effects", "Drug interactions", "Circumstances when caution is advisable"**, such as pregnancy, and **"Special precautions".** Another section sets out the **"Biological Systems supported"** and the botanical herb's **"Activities"** in the human body. **"Primary Applications", "Recommended Dosage", and "Key Active Constituents"** are also listed as well as a **"Clinical Reviews" and "Key Scientific References".**

NB. Many of the Phytonutrients included in the comprehensive Desktop Reference <u>target specific health needs</u>, which are not universal across the general population. Because the aim of this book is to address the <u>important universal reasons why everyone should supplement their diets</u>, it is not intended to go into the benefits of <u>all</u> the phyto-nutrients listed. Suffice it to say, there is likely to be an answer to many of the less common health issues people may want to address in the above Desktop Reference.

3rd PILLAR OF HEALTH – BONE NUTRIENTS.

The Food and Drug Authority (FDA) in the USA stated, *"In women over 65, the commonest cause of death is osteoporosis, more than heart disease and Cancer. Regular exercise and a healthy diet with enough calcium help teen, young adult Caucasian and Asian women and middle-aged women with a family history of the disease, maintain good bone health and may reduce their risk of osteoporosis later in life."*

Most People take their Bones for Granted – Bones are Living Human Tissue, <u>not</u> Metal Scaffolding!

The Key Bone Nutrients are Calcium and Magnesium (in the optimal 2:1 ratio) (see below under 4th Pillar of Health – Trace Elements – page 127), **Vitamin D3, Vitamin K, Boron, and Silicon.**

Vitamin D3 (ergocalciferol, cholecalciferol) helps maintain strong and healthy bones by retaining calcium, supports muscle strength and hearing.

Vitamin K (phylloquinone), apart from supporting healthy bones, controls blood clotting.

Boron is a mineral, which helps the body use calcium and may be beneficial for arthritis sufferers.

Silicon is another mineral, which is important for normal bone health.

4th PILLAR OF HEALTH – TRACE ELEMENTS AND MINERALS
(including Chelated Minerals & Metabolic Conditioners).

Our bodies also need trace amounts of minerals. We have all heard commercials about products containing Iron, Zinc, and Calcium. We also need Manganese, Copper, Iodine, Magnesium, Phosphorus, Chromium, and Molybdenum. As for Antioxidants, Selenium, Zinc, Copper, and Manganese top the list and were covered earlier in this book under the 1st Pillar of Health – Antioxidants – see page 80.

Minerals are "essential", meaning our bodies cannot produce them; they have to be obtained from our diet. Minerals, reacting with Enzymes to convert food into energy, are essential for growth to adulthood, and regulate all body processes such as movement, thinking, breathing, reproduction, muscles functioning etc. Minerals are involved in more body functions than any other basic nutrient that we consume, including, protein, vitamins, fats, carbohydrates, and water.

The minerals that we are very likely to be short of include the following:

NB. For information on the Four Important Antioxidant Minerals, Selenium, Zinc, Copper, and Manganese – see 1st Pillar of Health – Antioxidants (page 80).

Calcium, in addition to being a key bone nutrient, clots blood, contracts muscles, promotes healthy nerves, improves skin, bone and teeth health, relieves aching muscles, maintains correct acid/alkaline balance and reduces menstrual cramps and tremors.

Magnesium, in addition to being a key bone nutrient, strengthens teeth, promotes healthy muscles by helping them relax, so important for PMS, and for heart muscles and nervous system. Magnesium is essential for energy production and is involved as a co-factor in many enzymes in the body. <u>Calcium and Magnesium should be in the optimum 2:1 ratio</u>. Depletion of Magnesium can lead to asthma and cramps.

Chromium is a Metabolic Conditioner. It is part of the Glucose tolerance factor (GTF = Vitamin B3, glycine, glutamic acid & cystine + chromium). Chromium is the "starter motor" for insulin to balance blood sugar levels. It helps to normalise hunger and reduce cravings, improves lifespan, helps protect DNA and RNA, metabolises fat for energy whilst protecting lean muscle mass and is essential for heart function. Chromium works with the B-complex vitamins to assist in the body's metabolism of carbohydrates, protein, and fat for conversion into energy.

Iron is part of Haemoglobin in the blood, which transports oxygen and carbon dioxide to and from cells. Iron is a component of enzymes and is vital for energy production. Females require more iron than men and high levels of iron in men can lead to cardiovascular problems.

Molybdenum helps rid the body of the protein breakdown products, e.g. uric acid, strengthens teeth, and detoxifies the body from free radicals, petrochemicals, and sulphites.

Potassium enables nutrients to flow in and waste products to flow out of body cells. It promotes healthy nerves and muscles, maintains body fluid balance, relaxes muscles, helps secretion of insulin for blood sugar control to produce constant energy, is involved in metabolism, maintains the heart functioning and stimulates gut movements to encourage proper elimination. It is relatively easy to obtain sufficient potassium from our diets.

Vanadium helps make good use of glucose and supports metabolism.

Glucosamine is a building block for cartilage and connective tissue and is essential for supporting healthy joints. Many so-called arthritic conditions are due to a lack of good nutrition. Chondroitin is similar in chemical structure to Glucosamine and works broadly in the same way. Chondroitin is often found in "joint health products", usually with Glucosamine, but sometimes without it. You need to be aware that clinical studies indicate that no additional synergistic benefits result from combining Glucosamine and Chondroitin and for Chondroitin to be effective it needs to be from an expensive source, which is not the case with most of the Chondroitin products on the market. There are also many more clinical studies on the benefits of Glucosamine than there are on Chondroitin, and so best value for money is usually obtained from a Glucosamine based product without added Chondroitin.

Minerals Generally – The body cannot create Minerals; they have to be acquired. They are non-absorbable in their natural state; they're like tiny little rocks! Only if they are eaten with other particular foods, can the body absorb them and even then the natural "hit and miss combining" process is inefficient. The answer to ensuring minerals are effectively absorbed into the blood stream and on into the body cells, is "chelation", whereby an Amino Acid is wrapped around the mineral or metal, which makes the mineral highly absorbable. The minerals are then transported in the blood as a chelate, they cross the cell membrane as a chelate right into the cell where they catalyse enzyme reactions within the mitochondria in each cell. All energy in the human body comes from within the cell. Chelated Minerals give you Dynamic Energy!

Although some other mineral compounds such as citrates, gluconates, and lactates increase mineral absorption, in most cases they are less effective than chelates. Make sure that any minerals you consider taking are chelated!

5th PILLAR OF HEALTH – B VITAMINS.

The Key B Vitamins, which must all be in balance, are **B1** Thiamin, **B2** Riboflavin, **B3** Niacin, **B5** Pantothenic Acid, **B6** Pyridoxine, **B12** Cyanocobalamin, **Folic Acid** and **Biotin**. They are co-enzymes, which are principally involved in energy metabolic reactions. B Vitamins are water-soluble and so are not stored in the body in significant quantities. Therefore they are needed daily. The B complex of vitamins is closely inter-related, which means an inadequate intake of one impairs the utilisation of others. A deficiency of a single B vitamin is however relatively rare.

Vitamin B1 (Thiamin) is essential for energy production, brain function, and digestion. It helps the body make use of protein. It supports against depression, irritability, muscle weakness, and memory loss.

Vitamin B2 (Riboflavin) helps turn fat, sugars, and protein into energy. It is needed to repair and maintain healthy skin inside, especially mucous membranes, as well as on the surface of the skin. It helps to regulate body acidity and it is important for hair, nails, and eyes.

Vitamin B3 (Niacin) is essential for energy production, brain function and the skin. It helps balance blood sugar and lower cholesterol levels. It is also involved in inflammation and digestion.

Vitamin B5 (Pantothenic acid) is involved in energy production and controls fat metabolism. It is essential for brain and nerves. It helps to make anti-stress hormones (steroids such as cortisol). It maintains healthy skin and hair.

Vitamin B6 (Pyridoxine) is essential for protein digestion and utilisation, brain function and hormone production. It helps balance sex hormones, hence use in PMS and the menopause. It is a natural anti-depressant and diuretic. It helps control allergic reactions, supports restful sleep, and reduces damaging Homocysteine levels in the blood.

Vitamin B12 (Cyanocobalamin) is needed for making protein. It helps the blood carry oxygen; hence it is essential for energy. It is needed for synthesis of DNA and is essential for nerves. It also reduces damaging Homocysteine levels on the blood.

Biotin is particularly important in childhood. It helps the body use Essential Fats, assisting in promoting healthy skin, hair, nerves, and brain function.

Folic Acid / Folacin is critical during pregnancy, especially early-stage, for brain and nerve development and protects against neural tube defects in the unborn child. It is essential for brain and nerve function throughout life. It is needed for utilising protein and red blood cell formation. It also reduces damaging Homocysteine levels in the blood.

RESEARCH STUDIES ON B VITAMINS

Newsweek, USA reported on 11ᵗʰ August 1997 *"There has been a steady decline in Deaths from Heart Attacks, but Cholesterol levels haven't changed much... The reason for this deviation could be due to more control of **Homocysteine,** which is an Amino Acid, which plays a critical role in damaging arteries, and may be as significant as Smoking or Cholesterol."*

Homocysteine may cause the initial injury to the artery rather than cholesterol. *"Plasma total homocysteine levels are a strong predictor of mortality in patients with angiographically confirmed coronary artery disease."* – **Nygard et al. NEIM, 14ᵗʰ July 1997.**

Vitamins B6, B12, and Folic Acid reduce Homocysteine to safe levels. The minimum daily requirement of Folic Acid is 400 mcg for pre-menopausal women, especially a few months before and immediately after they become pregnant, in order to reduce the possibility of neural tube defects in unborn children.

6ᵗʰ PILLAR OF HEALTH – ESSENTIAL FATTY ACIDS

Fatty Acids are the basic building blocks of fats and oils. Contrary to popular myth, the body does need fat but it must be the right kind. Fatty Acids are called "Essential Fatty Acids (EFAs)" because they are essential to health and must be supplied through the diet. The body cannot create them. They are sometimes referred to as Vitamin F or Polyunsaturates.

There are Two Basic Categories of EFAs, designated "Omega-3" and "Omega-6". The average modern diet is substantially more deficient in Omega-3 Fatty Acids than in Omega-6s. Centuries ago when we were "hunter/gatherers", the ratio of our intake of Omega-3 Fatty Acids to Omega-6s, was the desirable Equal Ratio of 1:1. However, that Ratio has become very seriously out of balance over the last century and, believe it or not, is now 1:20 – Omega-3s to Omega-6s!

This is partly because the "grandmother" of the Omega-3 family, Linolenic Acid, and her metabolically active "children", EPA (Eicosapentaenoic Acid) and DHA (Docosahexaenoic Acid), from which Series 3 Prostaglandins are made, are more unsaturated and more prone to damage due to the heat in cooking and food processing than the "child", GLA (Gamma-Linoleic Acid) of the grandmother of the Omega-6 family, Linoleic Acid. This makes it easier to obtain sufficient Omega-6s from our diets. While Omega-6s provide health benefits, such as Evening Primrose Oil helping with PMS, it must be remembered that a high intake of Omega-6s could restrict the intake of Omega-3s. <u>It is therefore advisable to supplement just with Omega-3s</u> unless there are over-riding reasons why you need extra Omega-6s. <u>Every living cell in the body needs Essential Fatty Acids, which are critically important to the replication of all cells in the body. Out of balance Essential Fatty Acids can be damaging to the immune system</u>.

Series 3 Prostaglandins, which are derived from Omega-3 Fatty Acids, are essential for proper brain function, which affects vision, learning ability, coordination, and mood. They can help protect against and treat Mental Health conditions such as Dyslexia, Dyspraxia, Attention-Deficit/Hyperactivity Disorder (ADHD) and Schizophrenia. Prostaglandins are hormone like substances that act as chemical messengers and regulators of various body processes. Adequate levels of DHA are crucial to brain development, especially up to the age of 2, and EPA and DHA are crucial to brain performance throughout life.

Essential Fatty Acids are critical to maintaining good health in many other ways. They improve skin and hair, reduce blood pressure, lower cholesterol and triglyceride levels, reduce inflammation, help prevent arthritis, reduce the risk of blood clotting and support water balance.

The Principal Sources of Omega-3s are oily fish such mackerel, herring, tuna, anchovies and salmon, which are rich in EPA and DHA, plus linseed, hemp and pumpkin seeds.

The Principal Sources of Omega-6s, *(much less likely to be short of in your diet than Omega-3s)*, are Evening Primrose Oil and Borage oil, which are rich in Gamma-Linolenic Acid (GLA).

However, supplementing with pure Omega-3 products that are guaranteed free of contaminants is the safest way to ensure that you have a continuous, effective and safe intake of good quality Essential Omega-3 Fatty Acids, rather than eating a relatively large amount of oily fish on a regular basis, when you have no control over the source of the fish. As you may be aware, there is much concern globally about PCBs (Polychlorinated Biphenyls) and other pollutants that are found in oily fish, especially farmed fish and so this is one of those situations where supplementing could be more advisable than eating the "real thing!"

FINAL THOUGHTS ON YOUR SEARCH FOR DYNAMIC HEALTH

There is a rapidly increasing awareness amongst the population, that there <u>are</u> nutritional solutions to achieving Dynamic Health, which is being fuelled by the "Ageing of the Baby Boomers", who are searching for any way possible to hold onto their youth. What are they looking for? Answer – Dynamic Health – because they want to *"look good, feel good, perform better, keep away from disease, and die young as late as possible!"* Isn't that what you want?

At no other time in our history has the public interest in self-care and the use of natural health remedies been so widespread with more than 50% of the adult population of the US, Japan, and most of Europe consuming a dietary supplement on a regular basis. From these statistics it's clear that the acceptance of using dietary/nutritional supplements to promote health and reduce disease is here to stay.

So if you want to look good, feel good, perform better, keep away from disease and die young as late as possible, if you want to add life to your years, if you want to live better longer, you must be proactive!

Take charge of your health and supplement your diet twice daily with the best quality pharmaceutical grade multi-nutrient supplement you can get your hands on. Ideally, the supplement should be clinically proven in double-blind placebo controlled clinical studies on humans and made using pharmaceutical methodologies to ensure the highest standards of safety and efficacy. <u>"Twice daily" is important because most antioxidants only last in the blood for 12 hours</u>! In any case the body prefers its daily intake of food to come regularly throughout the day rather than mostly at one meal.

You should also make sure the multi-vitamin/mineral supplement you are considering contains comprehensive ranges of antioxidants, vitamins, chelated minerals, and phytonutrients to ensure you are covering all the first 5 Essential "Pillars of Health" – Antioxidants, Phytonutrients, Bone Nutrients, Trace Elements including Chelated Minerals and B-Vitamins. Due to the fragility of the Omega-3 Fatty Acids, for technical reasons, the 6th Pillar of Health – Essential Fatty Acids – is better supplied as a separate supplement on its own.

As Emerson said, *"The First Wealth in Life is Health"* – what is your health worth to you and your family – it's incalculable! Without good health you're nowhere. Taking a good quality multi-nutrient supplement, preferably proven through pharmaceutical methodologies for safety and efficacy, every day, is the best health insurance policy you and your family could ever take out, provided you combine it with exercise and a well balanced diet, you keep away from tobacco and moderate your intake of alcohol! Taking supplements is like taking out an insurance policy; there are no guarantees. In any case we are all different, with each one of us having our own biochemical makeup.

Remember, many of us eat the wrong things. We eat what is appealing to the palate but not satisfying to the immune system. We are simply not supplying our bodies with the nutrients, especially antioxidants, which they need in order to keep the body in balance to protect us against diseases and enable us to enjoy continuous Dynamic Health.

But as you will have gathered from this book, leading scientists across the world have proved that there is something that we can do to avoid taking unnecessary risks with our health through being malnourished and immune deficient, even though many people do not appreciate that they are.

If you are committed to achieving Dynamic Health you should:

Look at your lifestyle habits and commit to change them where necessary.

Start taking appropriate exercise if you're not exercising vigorously for at least 30 minutes, 3 times a week.

Consider any changes to your diet that would be advisable and

Start taking a "twice-a-day" multi-vitamin/mineral/micronutrient supplement plus a separate Omega-3 product twice-a-day.

But you do need to remember – not all supplements are created equal! Do make sure, by asking the supplier whether the manufacturer of the supplement you are considering buying can prove its safety and efficacy. Ideally it should be made to pharmaceutical standards to enable it to be consistent, tablet-to-tablet, and capsule-to-capsule and to be guaranteed to conform to the contents declared on the label, which is far from the case for many products on the market, according to independent studies. Also, the supplement you choose should, ideally, be supported by clinical studies on humans, which will go a long way towards indicating the benefits you could expect from the supplement.

Make sure you ask those questions, as they will have an important bearing on your future health!

.... *And one final point!*

When you receive answers to the above questions as to whether the multivitamin/mineral/micronutrient supplement you are considering is made to pharmaceutical standards and is clinically proven on humans, you would still be depending on third party information, i.e. trials on other people. <u>You would still not be able to prove that the product you choose actually delivers the nutrients it should into your own body!</u>

But only recently – that has all changed!

The final section in this book should be extremely interesting to you because it is revolutionising human health and nutrition!

BIO-PHOTONIC SCANNER

I'm sure you will be interested to know that only recently it has become possible to measure the level of antioxidant protection in your own body tissue in a non-invasive and convenient way in "real time", i.e. in just three minutes! This is known as your "antioxidant score"! A series of your antioxidant scores at say 4-weekly intervals from when you start taking a supplement will show how you are benefiting from that supplement, conclusively proving that the Antioxidants in the Supplement are actually getting to the "Site of Action" in your body tissues, where Free Radicals and Antioxidants battle it out – assuming, of course, the supplement is of sufficient quality.

This new technology was developed by the University of Utah in the U.S.A., and is called the BioPhotonic Scanner, which uses a laser to measure antioxidant levels in human skin. *(This doesn't mean the laser drills a hole in your skin!)* The BioPhotonic Scanner uses Nobel Prize – Winning Raman Spectroscopy, which emits a unique low light laser to scan the palm of your hand to measure the level of carotenoid antioxidants present at what is known as the "site of action", which is the holy grail for measuring a nutritional bio-marker. It's completely painless, accurate, and convenient. Carotenoids are scientifically proven to be an excellent indicator of your overall antioxidant status in your body, i.e. the level of protection against free radical oxidative damage you have in your body.

Carotenoids are very representative of the total antioxidant defence network in the body. This has been shown in many clinical studies including those conducted by **Prof. Lester Packer**, who is known in medical circles across the world as **"The Father of Antioxidant Theory"** and is the foremost Scientist who has been researching Free Radicals and Antioxidants for the last 40 years. Antioxidants do not exist in isolation - they are intimately linked together insofar that if one breaks, the whole antioxidant network is weakened. Carotenoids act as Sentinels to this Network and are the first line of defence. <u>Measuring Carotenoid tissue concentration is clinically proven to be a very effective way of monitoring overall antioxidant health.</u>

Prior to the BioPhotonic Scanner, the only option available to measure the antioxidant status of the body was to cut out a chunk of skin, grind it up, and measure what was found! Few people would be willing to subject themselves to such a method on a regular basis! Blood tests and urine tests do not measure at the "site of action"; they take time and are inconvenient. Blood tests are also invasive and influenced by postprandial fluctuations, i.e. they are affected by recent meals etc.

It has also been proved to world-leading Scientific Organisations such as the New York Academy of Sciences, Oxygen Club of California, several members of the "Federation of American Societies for Experimental Biology" (FASEB), the American Society of Nutritional Sciences, Gordon Research Conference, American Society of Clinical Nutrition and the American College of Nutrition that when Carotenoids are increased in the diet, these substances initially accumulate in the lipoproteins in blood (Smidt et al.1999). This increase is then reflected in an increase in the Carotenoid concentration in all organs in the body, which can take up lipoproteins, including the skin. <u>Thus the direct measurement of Carotenoids in skin provides information about their levels at "sites of action" all over the body. This is a distinct advantage over measurements of Carotenoids in blood plasma.</u>

A Paper entitled *"Nutritional Significance and Measurement of Carotenoids", published in the Peer-reviewed Journal – Current Topics in Nutraceutical Research (May 2004)* showed that BioPhotonic Scanner Antioxidant Scores correlate favourably with Blood Antioxidant Scores. The paper examined the role of Carotenoids in cell, eye, cardiovascular, skin, prostate and general health and reiterated the overall antioxidant function, which is to neutralise free radicals. Dr. Carsten R. Smidt, Ph.D., FACN, Vice President of Global Research and Development and Doug Burke, Ph.D., Research Scientist at Pharmanex, published the review that emphasises the benefits of the BioPhotonic Scanner.

"This Paper summarises everything a scientist would want to know about Carotenoids and the Scanner", stated Dr. Smidt. *"This new and effective way of measuring Carotenoids can be used in clinical studies to validate reported nutrient and vegetable intake data, which is*

notoriously unreliable. In addition, the Scanner Assesses the Body's Antioxidant Status. Antioxidants have profound health benefits that have been documented in tens of thousands of clinical studies, and knowing your personal antioxidant status will help you eat and live better."

Perhaps one of the most exciting findings of this paper was that Scanner Antioxidant scores correlate favourably with Blood Antioxidant Scores. *"The blood test to measure Carotenoids is the old gold standard,"* noted Dr. Smidt. *"Our findings show that the BioPhotonic Scanner is rapidly becoming a New and Better Standard. The Scanner makes it possible for Carotenoid and Overall Antioxidant Status in the General Population to be measured, which has never been possible before."*

"Everyone should use the BioPhotonic Scanner to learn their Optimal Body Defence Score. Once you have your number, work to increase it and maintain it with a diet rich in fruits, vegetables and vitamin supplements." Dr. Lester Packer. CNN Money, 17th Sept.2002.

CONCLUSION

It is hoped that this book has gone some way in assisting you in your Search for Dynamic Health and that it has helped you to appreciate and understand the enormous health benefits that we can all derive from supplementing our diets.

What is more, now that you can measure the benefits to your health of your diet and the supplements you are taking; it makes even more sense to take supplements.

We eat the wrong things. We eat what is appealing to the palate but not satisfying to the immune system. We're simply not supplying our bodies with the nutrients that they need to protect us against diseases and to slow up the ageing process. **But all that can change because there is a revolution happening out there right now.**

It has long been said in medical circles that putting balance into the body and feeding it with a broad spectrum of antioxidants would revolutionise the face of modern medicine, but without a reliable, convenient and painless way of measuring antioxidant levels, that revolution was destined to never get off the ground! With the recent development of the BioPhotonic Scanner, that Antioxidant Revolution is now taking off!

You've taken the first step towards Dynamic Health by investing your time to read this book.

You've started down the road towards better health and ultimately a better and more fulfilling life. Now it remains up to you.

Will you reflect on the knowledge you've gained from this book and achieve your ambition of enjoying continuous Dynamic Health for the rest of your life?

Will you be proactive and modify your diet and lifestyle choices, where appropriate, and supplement your diet with important nutrients and a broad spectrum of antioxidants?

WILL YOU JOIN THE NEW REVOLUTION?